# LOOK BETTER
# FEEL BETTER
# LIVE BETTER

by
## Elizabeth Roddick

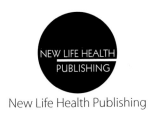

New Life Health Publishing

NEW LIFE HEALTH PUBLISHING
43 Newlands Road, Newlands, Glasgow G43 2JH, United Kingdom

First published in Great Britain in 2005 by NEW LIFE HEALTH PUBLISHING

10 9 8 7 6 5 4 3 2

First Edition

© 2005 Elizabeth Roddick and NEW LIFE HEALTH PUBLISHING

Elizabeth Roddick asserts the moral right to be the author of this work.

A catalogue record for this book is available from the British Library

ISBN-10: 0-9551461-0-0
ISBN-13: 978-0-9551461-0-7

CONDITIONS OF SALE
This book is sold subject to the condition that it shall not, by way of trade or otherwise,
be lent, re-sold, hired out or otherwise circulated without the publisher's prior consent in
any form of binding or cover other than that in which it is published and without a similar
condition including this condition being imposed on the subsequent purchaser.

The contents of this book do not fall within the terms of any blanket copyright provisions
that may be granted by any other publisher.

Permission for the reproduction of any item in this book must be sought from the
individual copyright holder.

Permission for the reproduction of the typesetting of any item

## DEDICATION

*This book is dedicated to my husband
who supports me through all my endeavours,
my mother who, almost totally blind, with her indomitable spirit,
continues to strive in all her adversity
and to my late brother who may not have died prematurely of cancer
if he had been aware of the importance of lifestyle in prevention.*

## ACKNOWLEDGEMENTS

*My husband, Douglas Roddick. My brother Mike Ure, Focus Marketing.*
*Gavin Bonnar, Chameleon Design (the original book designer).*
*Don Cunningham at Westcoast Graphics,*
*Will Springer, Deputy Editor at www.scotsman.com.*
*Dr. John Maclean, Medical Director, The National Stadium Sports Medicine*
*Centre, Hampden Park Glasgow.*
*Julie Hanson, The Chi Yoga Centre Glasgow,*
*Shelley Banks of Shelbyfit. Ian Pollock, The Silva Method,*
*Bill McCluskie, Linda Harrower, Margaret Lethrie.*
*Pat Martin. Anne Hall, Anthony Robbins,*
*Dr. Surji Virk, Piers Whitney, Carla MacKenzie, Professor Alexander Wedderburn,*
*Patricia Hay, Senior Vocal Tutor at the Royal Academy of Music and Drama.*

Photograph of young boy fascinated by water (Page 69) is Euan McGillivray
Hydrotherapy photograph (page 74) by kind permission of Jordan Harboldt,www.sensationalspas.biz
Seaweed photograph (page 75) is by kind permission of www.bariez.com.
Kirlian photographs (page 84) are by kind permission of Christopher Wodtke.
T'ai Chi photograph (page 104) by kind permission of Inger Johanne Vesje, www.taichitunsberg.com
Climbing photograph (page 112) by kind permission of Douglas Cunningham.
Concorde photo (page 127) copyright Art Brett

# CONTENTS

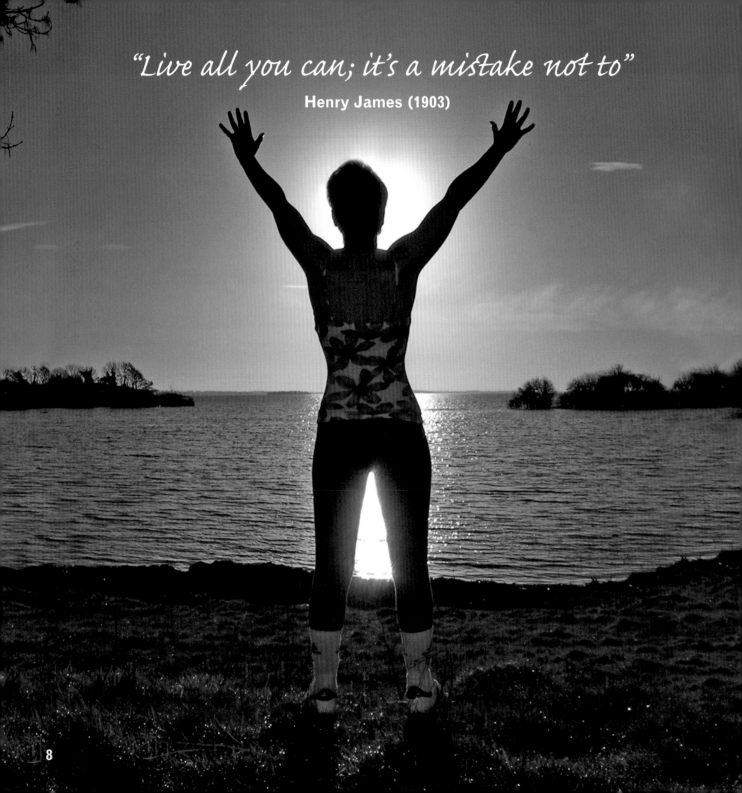

"Live all you can; it's a mistake not to"

Henry James (1903)

# INTRODUCTION

Get yourself in front of a mirror. Take a long hard look and make a decision.
Do you want to look the same, feel the same and be living the same life
in one year's time?

If your answer is "No", then you will find this book a useful guide to moving
yourself from your current baseline. To be realistic, you must look from where
you are starting.

A small shift can make a huge difference to the way you feel, look or go about your
daily activities. You must decide what you want.

Once you have made that commitment in writing, make some decisions on how
responsible you are going to be for living your life to the fullest.

Many people make New Year resolutions about changing lifestyle.
They take their habit smoking or overeating, for example… decide to stop doing
the thing they know is wrong and, for a short time, are extremely successful in that
change. What happens a few weeks later is, they revert back to the old way of life.
That makes them feel like a failure and they may say, "well, that's life I suppose".

What about your own life?
Are there things in your life that need to be changed?
If you want a fantastic life then you should have a plan.

Plot your life on the chart right now-the **Star of Life Plan** (See next page and
further information page)
0% is the worst possible scenario and 100% is your idea of fulfilment.

There is another Star of Life Plan at the back of this book. Plot where you would like
to be, read the examples I give and look at the relevant steps to help you move
forward towards fulfilling your Life Plan.

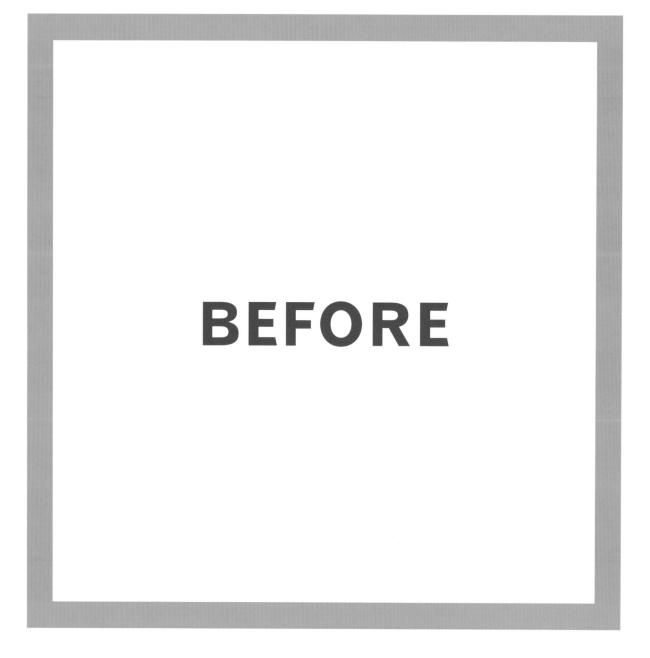

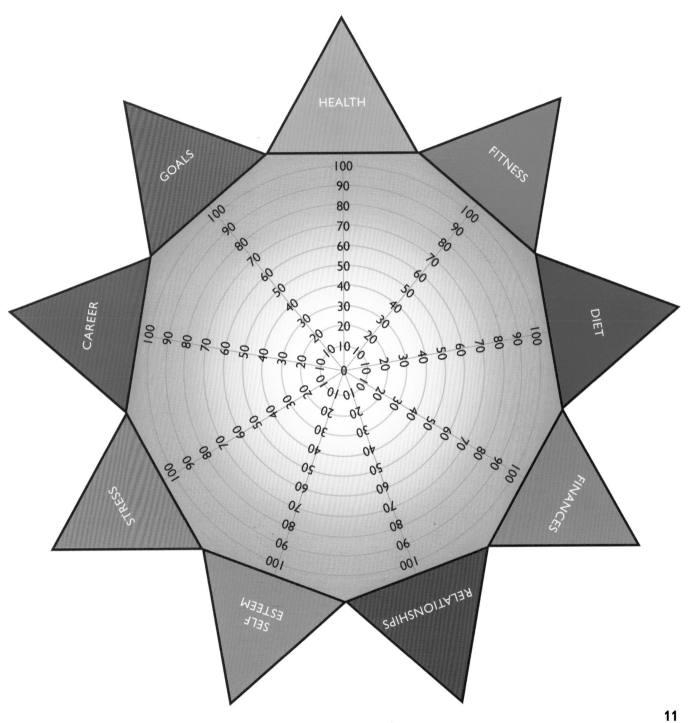

# INTRODUCTION

This book looks at **lasting** change.

If you're feeding your body the wrong type of fuel--whether its your diet, lack of exercise or your relationships-- then, you're not going to feel as good as you should. I know you will find something in the following pages that touches your inner self, makes you feel alive and moves you to a higher level of achievement.

I started this journey to improve my own well-being because I believe we don't have to prematurely age.There are races in the world where the people live dynamic, vital lives well into their eighties, nineties and beyond. For many Westerners, growing old is an inevitable decline of both our physical and mental capacities and this results in a poor quality of life.

This doesn't have to be… **if we change our attitude to ageing.**

Your age can be expressed in different ways, for example your biological age can be as much as 15 years younger than your chronological age. *(See Markers of our Biological Age on the following page.)*

This "reduction" in terms of your age may be achieved by following the steps in this book only if you have a total belief in the process.

You then need to make these steps a way of life. The only way to change things for the better is to believe you can do **and believe in yourself.**

Everyone has a unique potential but it's easy to become diverted by life's trials and tribulations and to let everyday life get in the way. If you can discover your unique contribution to the world and then follow that path, the reward is true inner peace.

The author wishes to point out that the ten-point plan reflects her own life- changing experience and she does not accept any responsibility for anyone following this path without seeking the appropriate professional advice if required.

# MARKERS OF OUR BIOLOGIGAL AGE

- Aerobic capacity

- Antioxidant levels

- Auditory acuity

- Blood pressure

- Blood glucose control

- Body fat

- Bone density

- Cholesterol and lipid levels

- Hormone levels

- Immune function

- Metabolic activity

- Muscle mass and strength

- Skin thickness

- Temperature regulation

- Visual acuity

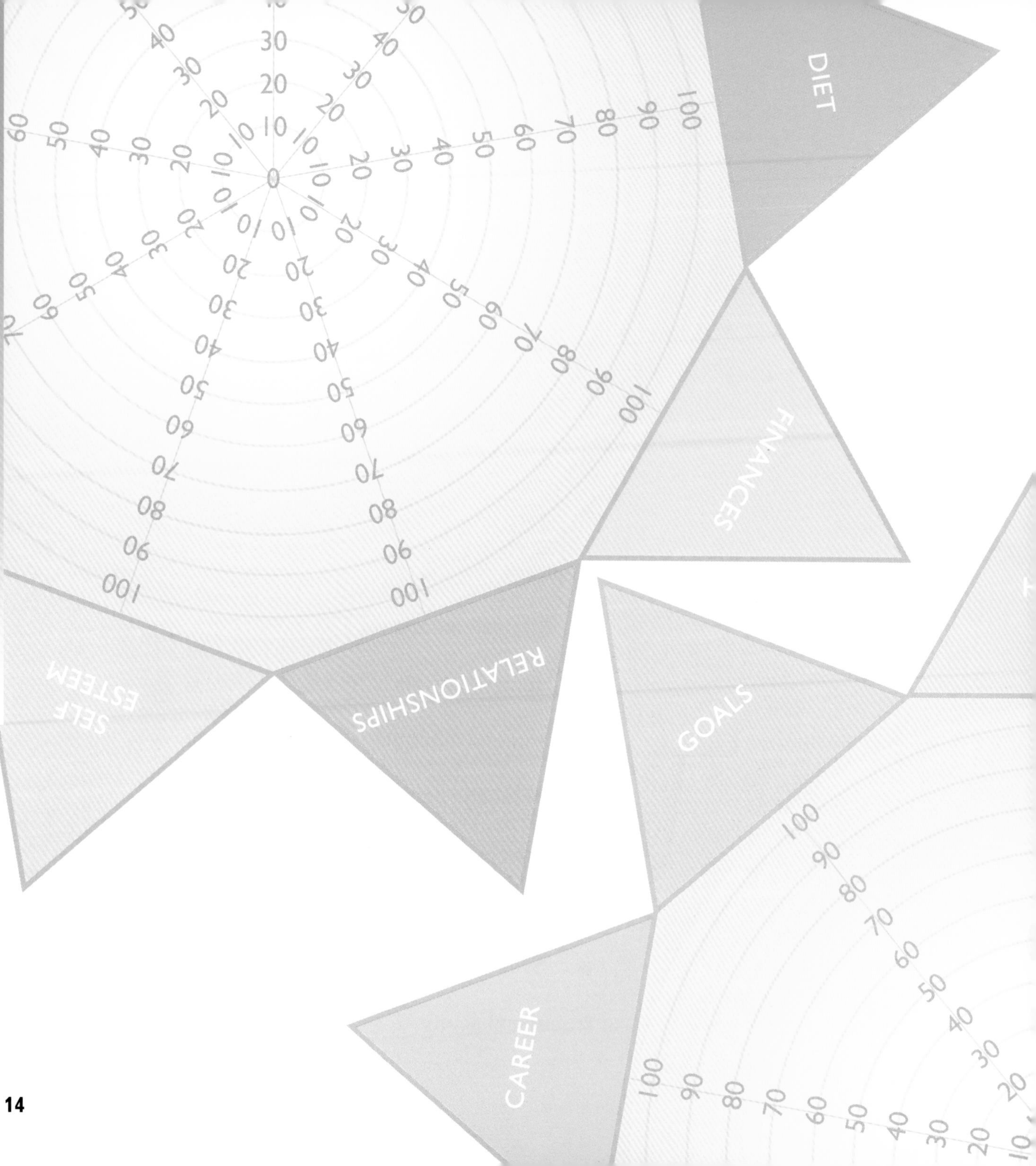

DIET

FINANCES

RELATIONSHIPS

SELF ESTEEM

GOALS

CAREER

100 90 80 70 60 50 40 30 20

# STAR OF LIFE

*The purpose of the Star of Life is as a tool to assist you in measuring the quality of your life at any given point. The following chapters are intended to provide you with the information to help you make improvements. It is important to note that although some of these chapter headings and colour codes are similar to certain Star of Life sections, they are not to be taken as interchangeable.*

How much time have you spent planning your life? I bet you've spent more time planning your holidays! If you want a fantastic life then you have to plan it.

How would you feel if you woke up every morning crackling with ideas, knowing that you were moving ahead towards your ultimate goals? When you start planning your life, things will start to happen. It's like a missile that has been launched, propelling you to where you want to go with all the enrichment of life's experiences on the journey.

Have you ever helped someone in the past and years later something happens which repays the kindness in a totally different way? Some people call it coincidences which, when you look back, have helped you manifest many of your dreams. I'll give you an example of what I mean.

A young man called John was trying to get his business off the ground. It was a restaurant and he had spent a long time refurbishing the building, meeting all the criteria for food hygiene standards and producing small but interesting menus so that when he finally opened his doors he expected a rush of curious people to his business. When John first opened few people decided to try out his restaurant and, despite advertising in the local press, he was struggling to keep the business going.

One day a man walked into the restaurant and, after ordering his meal, asked John if he remembered meeting him several years ago. John couldn't think where he had seen him before. As the man talked John began to visualise the scene where he had helped a homeless person who had literally fallen into the gutter. John helped the man to his feet and took him to a nearby hostel where he was given food and shelter. Unbelievably, this was the same man, well dressed, obviously well off and here to help John all he could.

# STAR OF LIFE

Simon Black was the man's name and he recounted to John that that act of kindness had somehow triggered a thought in his head. Simon began to look at his life and realised he didn't want to stay as a "down and out" and asked the staff in the hostel for help. Luckily one of the staff knew of a charity that helped disadvantaged people get back into employment.

Gradually Simon began to get his life back together and he could start to see the potential in working hard and moving forward. His business grew from his love of the stage and he developed several groups of itinerant entertainers who could perform short plays or medleys of songs in any venue, no matter how small. This business, said Simon, was thriving and he was here today to pay John back for helping him when it was most needed.

Simon then offered John some of his acts at reduced prices and contacts with the press so that John's restaurant would begin to have the reputation of an enjoyable night out with great variety. Before long, John was so financially secure that he was able to pay off his bank loan, employ extra staff and even have some time off at weekends.

You see, to realise the future you want you need to help more and more people get what they want and be mindful that everyone you meet needs to be treated with respect. The more people you help, the greater will be your reward--not just financially but spiritually as well. It also means a great deal more when the act of kindness is done with no expectation of thanks.

But back to the life plan. When you're aimlessly just getting through each day, you feel unfulfilled, lacking in energy and depressed.

Someone who has a purpose in life is young, vibrant and full of energy. So let's get planning your life!

# STAR OF LIFE

First, I want you to look at the Star of Life illustration and I'll talk you through how to use it.

The topics I've chosen might not fit exactly with your aspirations so feel free to change one or two so that you feel ownership of the plan.

One lady I know wanted to have spirituality instead of finances because while reasonably wealthy she had not found an inner peace that can come with spiritual belief.

It's necessary, however to keep the topic of health, because your health is often *the* most important factor in relation to the other topics in the Star of Life -- career, fitness, finances, relationships etc..

The next thing to do is to start plotting your present status.
Say your finances are not in very good order, then you could put a mark at 20% of what they should be.

On the other hand, if you have a brilliant career you could say you are at 90% of your potential--congratulations, by the way!

Go around the whole star thinking about where you are at the moment with regard to each topic.

Mark a cross at the percentage and join up all the crosses.

(100% is the best you could be and 0% is your worst in terms of your potential.)

FITNESS

100
90
80
70
60
50

# STAR OF LIFE

I've given you an example of someone's initial chart.

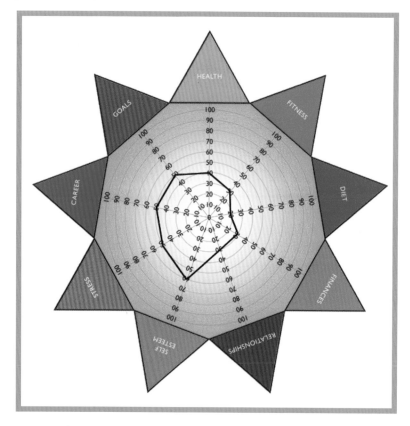

This person had a few challenges to overcome which he worked on.

What does your chart look like?

You need to start on one topic that you know would make a difference to your life if you had exactly what you wanted in that area.

I'm going to start to work through the example of finances.
There are a series of questions that you need to answer.

# STAR OF LIFE

## FINANCES

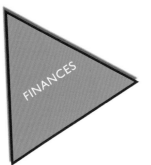

1. What do you want? Write down exactly how much you need to earn in order to have the lifestyle that you want.

2. How would you feel if you had all the money you needed?
   What difference would it make to yourself and your family?
   You need to write down all the good things that would happen when you reach your goal. You need to have great reasons for pursuing this goal. Now, how does that make you feel?

3. What sort of person do you need to become to achieve that goal?
   Do you need to practice generosity every day to make your financial goal happen? What about discipline? Do you have that characteristic now?

4. What would happen if you didn't achieve the financial goal you desire? People automatically move away from pain. Take the example of when you accidentally put your hand near a fire. What are the painful consequences of not achieving? Would you be unfulfilled? Would it mean that other people around you might suffer?
   This is another way of propelling you towards your financial dreams.

5. What do you have to do to get there? What would you need to do to earn the money you eventually require for your ultimate lifestyle?

6. Now, take what you have to do and divide it into steps. Each step needs to have a daily *"to do"* factor. By that I mean, each day you have to do something to move yourself forward along the right path.

7. You have to enjoy your journey! That's why step 2 above is there.

STAR OF LIFE

STEP ONE

Keep referring back to how you are going to feel when you experience the fruits of your labour. You need to have exciting reasons for pursuing this goal everyday.

In 1953, at Yale University, those leaving were asked if they had set written goals for their lives and plans to accomplish them. Of those graduating that year, only 3% admitted to having done so. In 1973, the surviving members of the class were interviewed again, and astonishingly, the 3% who had set written goals with plans were worth more in financial terms than the entire 97% put together.

Interestingly enough, Jack Zufelt who has written the programme *"The Power of Desire,"* feels that writing down goals are a waste of time.

What is important, in his opinion, is desire. You have to make up your own mind on that one but certainly, if you don't desire anything then no amount of writing down goals and plans are going to help manifest the future you want.

You have to ask yourself how you feel about money? We often hear the saying *"money is the root of all evil"*, but it is in fact the love of money that causes problems. If money is central to your life, you pursue it before anything or anyone else and you will be out of balance.

Not many people, as they reach the end of their life, think purely of money matters.

Most people realise what has been important in their lives and it generally has to do with relationships, family and friends.

# STAR OF LIFE

You will probably have heard of the 10% rule. If you save 10% of everything you earn, you will eventually become financially independent.

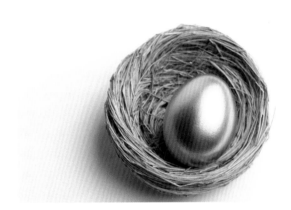

One definition of this could be if you stopped work, you would not need to worry about your financial future.

Try to put an amount of money away regularly in a secure place like a bank or building society.

Every week or month try to add to this fund. If you can keep adding regular amounts (and resist touching it) your savings will continue to grow in size.

The secret to being financially independent is to always pay this account first, use the rest for expenses and have something left over for investing or giving to charity.

You can't spend everything you earn because when you start borrowing, particularly with credit cards, you are just losing money on a downward spiral.

It's also a good idea to become knowledgeable about investing your money.
You only have to look at the pop stars that have lost millions through hiring people who mismanaged their funds. These stars didn't keep themselves informed and didn't ask the right questions of their advisors.

An interesting concept concerning having enough money for the future is that of "multiple streams of income". By that I mean not having just one income from a regular job but even earning money while you sleep.

Websites, of course, are a way of promoting products or services at any time of the day.

# STAR OF LIFE

Another idea is *"network marketing"*.

Donald Trump was asked if there was anything he would do differently if he had his time over again. His reply was that he would go into network marketing.
Someone in the audience guffawed and Trump looked directly at him and said:

> *"That's why I'm up here and you're down there."*

So what is network marketing? Simply, it is about introducing people to products that you are both using and are enthusiastic about and they in turn introduce others who then use the products, and so on.

The analogy is, if you introduced someone to a restaurant then every time they used that restaurant you would receive a commission. They, in turn, might introduce someone else to that restaurant and at that point both you and your "down liner" would receive a commission.

Can you imagine being rewarded every time you introduced someone to that restaurant and these restaurants were all over the country? The person you first recommended to visit that particular restaurant knew others who then used the restaurant and referred others and so on and you got paid every time all those people went to these restaurants for as long as you live.

Thousands of people in this country earn significant secondary or even primary incomes with network marketing. If you want to know more refer to the information page at the back of the book.

Your attitude toward money is important and relates to how much money you have at present.

People who denigrate those having money and think it is wrong to be in that position will always be poor. When you do have more money than you require, then that is when you look outside your own life.

# STAR OF LIFE

Many wealthy people-- who, incidentally, usually provide work for scores of people and whose taxes give government the resource to help those less fortunate-- have started charity funds in order to give something back into the society that has helped them become a financial success.

Dennis Stevenson is the author of *"Your Genius and Money"* and has taught the *"Money Workshop"* in San Francisco over the last twenty years. He has developed the theory that money is a symbol or a physical sign of the flow or management of our lives.

You have to examine your life and see where the flow has stopped. It could be that your tax return is late or something such as a relationship with a family member is troubling you.

You have to sort out the stoppages in your life before you can expect money to flow in. The analogy Dennis gives us is that of a bucket of muddy water in the desert, representing the state of your life, and someone comes along with an ice-cold pitcher of water representing opportunities. Would you want them to empty the pitcher of water into your bucket of muddy water?

Examine your life and clear up the things you have been putting off.
Clarity brings a release and an ability that moves you towards the amount of money you want to acquire. Sort out what is not moving or is stuck in your physical world for you to attract wealth.

Once you have completed the tidying up exercise then decide what you want and plan the next steps to get there. Always concentrate on the positive result as if you have already achieved your goal rather than entertain thoughts of failure.

# STAR OF LIFE

In order that you can achieve the financial standard you wish you need to find people that you can help with their goals.

They will be eager to help and soon you will find yourself moving quickly in the direction of your dreams.

No one has complete control of their finances without first giving the greatest possible service to others.

What value can you add in pursuit of your financial goal that people will recognise and be eager to pursue?

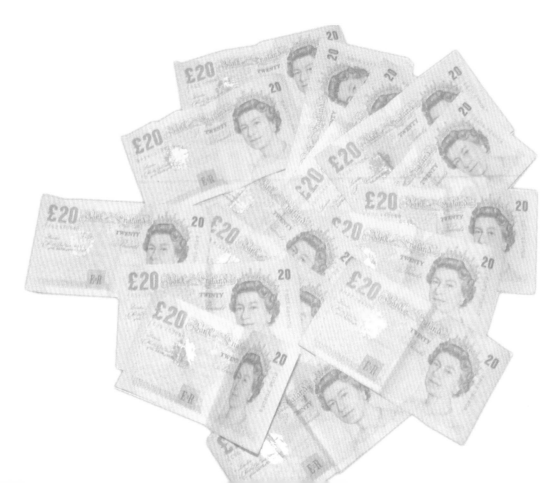

# STAR OF LIFE

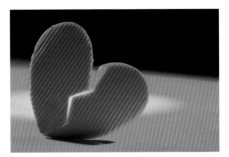

## RELATIONSHIPS

Relationships can shape the quality of your life. They are so important that it is worthwhile mentioning in this section while relating them to the Star of Life.

Read the section on self-esteem because to create a warm, rewarding and exciting relationship with someone else, you have to have an equivalent relationship with yourself.

What do I mean by that? Louise Hay is a metaphysical lecturer and teacher and the best selling author of eighteen books. Her audiotape programme "*The Power is within You*" expands on the philosophy *"loving the self"* by promoting the concept of allowing yourself to be deserving of what's good in your life. Also, Hay endorses praising yourself because, in her words, "when you berate yourself you belittle the power that created you." You were meant to love yourself so don't think there is anything wrong with that if it feels uncomfortable.

As always, look at your own score in terms of a significant other. Do you have a 0% score because you have never been in a serious relationship but want to be? If your score is around 40-50%, are you in the right relationship but have got to a stage where each person is taking the other for granted or is it boring?

**RELATIONSHIPS**

Karen had so much fun with the star because she wanted to find her soul mate. She plotted her score as 15% because she had been without a "significant other" for most of her adult life. She was now almost 40.

*(In the chapter on relationships I suggest that you visualise your ideal mate, what he or she would look like and what sort of characteristics would that person have?)*

Karen found this easy to do, but I had to point out that she had to look at herself when compiling the list because her "ideal" person needs to be attracted to her characteristics.

25

# STAR OF LIFE

We all know that someone who marries the "boy next door" who has similar values, beliefs and wealth tends to have sustainable relationships. In the first flush of love, people look for excitement and fulfilment and don't tend to focus on the real differences in fundamental values.

For example, if you are truly a family person and the love of your life wants to live an itinerant existence touring the world, then sooner or later it's not going to work.

The key to finding the right person is to spend some time thinking about the values and beliefs this person has to have. In other words if these characteristics were not present, then there was no point in continuing with the relationship.

This was the great thing about Karen's position. She took the time to prepare before making another monumental mistake. (In years gone by Karen had attracted partners that when she looks back now were unsuitable, not being congruent with her fundamental beliefs and values.)

So where was she going to find this fun-loving, gregarious dancer?
It certainly wasn't going to be at the funeral directors' annual meeting!

Karen looked around at the sort of hobbies and activities that she liked to do and plumped on joining a Salsa dance class and an amateur drama club that specialised in an enormous chorus with many people of all ages, men and women.

That day, she made two phone calls, one to the dance club and the other to the theatrical group. She was now going out socialising every Tuesday and Thursday.

During the next few months Karen met lots of people, and just for fun she would reflect on the important values she had to have in a relationship to see how they compared. In the past she would have dated some of her new friends but this time she knew exactly what she wanted and eventually, yes, Gordon appeared as a new member of the dance club.

# STAR OF LIFE

At first he appeared too reserved to be her type, but by the time he got around to asking her out after dancing with her for a few weeks she realised just how much alike they were. This relationship did develop and several weeks later she realised that their values and beliefs were about the same.

Actually, some other characteristics that she hadn't written down including surprising her by turning up or giving her little gifts unexpectedly were present which Karen had never experienced in a relationship before. She loved the attention and eventually realised she loved Gordon.

Did they have disagreements? Of course they did but because the underlying beliefs, values and characteristics were similar they soon worked out their differences.

If you can identify with Karen's circumstances, I hope you can see how this works. Planning what she actually wanted meant there was less chance of disappointment.

Karen also spent some time reflecting on why some of her earlier relationships had failed.

One reason is often because the person continues to feel and act the same way a second time.

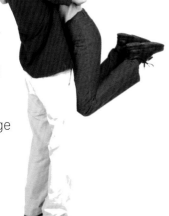

They wonder why the relationship is falling apart one year down the line but if they look at the pattern of their own behaviour and the fact that they disagree on fundamental beliefs, no wonder the relationship is struggling.

What about yourself? Are there behaviours you can change of yourself to make things better? Assuming you can "fix" something basic in a partner's nature can lead to resentment that ultimately leads to arguments. Learning to accept what you can't change and becoming more alike a partner can improve relationships greatly.

# STAR OF LIFE

I'll give you an example of this.

Mary had always hated her husband Bill smoking and used to nag him about the health problems-- she didn't want to lose him prematurely. Smoking is obviously a way of meeting some need that isn't being met in an alternative way.

Rather than continuing to nag, Mary thought of the reasons why Bill smoked and tried to empathise rather than always criticise. Bill used smoking mainly to relax and reduce the stress he built up from his work.

Mary looked around at classes for relaxation and gave him a year's subscription to a class as a birthday gift. She knew he probably wouldn't go on his own, so she bought her own subscription and went along as well. Yes, he did eventually give up smoking.

More importantly, Mary's change in attitude and the fact that both were taking part in activities helped them become closer as a couple.

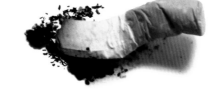

Sylvia and Tom were coming up for their 20th year in marriage. Just for a lark (or so they thought) they scored themselves on the Star of Life grid.

A score of 0% meant the marriage was over and 100% was where they had the most fulfilling, passionate, exciting relationship anyone could imagine.

Each of them was a little hesitant to show their scores since they were pretty low; things were predictable. They had got used to each other and there wasn't much excitement in their lives. I'm sure you can imagine a couple just like this.
So, what happened?

# STAR OF LIFE

The first thing they both did individually was to decide what sort of relationship each wanted. They answered the following questions:

1. Does your partner have to have a great sense of humour or do you prefer someone with a more serious disposition?

2. What about being able to share in a totally open way?

3. How important is it to have complete trust in your partner?

4. How do you feel when your partner praises you?
   Is it important to be praised and acknowledged or not?

5. How much quality time do you spend with each other?
   *By quality time I don't mean sitting in the same room with the television on!*

6. Do you go away together, just as a couple without friends and family?

By answering these questions, Tom and Sylvia started to understand the needs of the other partner and could move towards fulfilling those needs. Also, they began to realise the time element in their relationship. If you are too busy working-- or mainly out separately with your own friends-- then the relationship is bound to suffer.

Since they both wanted the relationship to get better they were willing to change how they related to each other and how much time each of them gave to the relationship. Sylvia realised that she never really praised Tom for the way he helped her with her work, the house and a family problem that meant she had to go away at least every fortnight. Tom on the other hand never encouraged Sylvia to bring out the feminine fun-loving side of her nature.

That is one of the key tasks to do. Think back to when you first met.
What were the things that really excited you about your other half?

# STAR OF LIFE

Have the years meant that you have inadvertently suppressed the qualities that first attracted you to each other? If you can start to unearth these qualities then I can guarantee that things will start to improve. It did for Tom and Sylvia.

What if you have done this exercise and realise that you're actually in the wrong relationship--your Star of Life percentage is around the 5% mark?

If you're honest, you're probably hanging in there *"because of the children"* or *"because of the security"* angle. The first thing to do is to ask yourself *"do I seriously want to make this relationship better?"* You can move a 5% score on the scale to 90% by employing some of the steps I have mentioned.

If, for example, you married when you were very young, then it may be that you have matured into a totally different person. Your outlook on life has changed dramatically and your partner has stayed the same.

You have to ask the question is the difference fundamental or can you change? Does your partner feel the same about altering his or her outlook or beliefs? If the answer to these difficult questions is that change is not feasible, then you have to seriously consider asking yourself -- does this relationship deserve my full attention?

As I said at the beginning of this section, an outstanding relationship with your partner can shape the quality of your life and can be obtained if you let him or her know how special they are to you.

If you make your partner feel as if they are the most important person around, they will want to please you and will want to play a significant role in your life.

Aim for 100% on the scale.

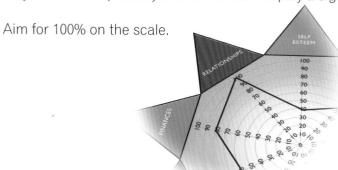

# STAR OF LIFE

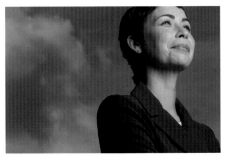

## SELF-ESTEEM

Have you ever noticed when someone comes into a room full of people (I'll use the female gender on this occasion), the person who has a high self-esteem looks relaxed and confident? She knows she looks good and therefore her outer appearance portrays that feeling.

People don't just acquire this feeling overnight; they have to have an inner confidence that comes from how they feel about themselves.

Loving yourself means that you can give love unreservedly to others.

Let's look at your own percentage. Do you think you have low self-esteem or high? Put a cross between 0%, which means basically your dead or 100% where you never have any doubts about how you feel, look or whether you can do a particular task. Most people are about 60%, but may be your score is lower so let's start with that scenario.

What is the reason your self-esteem is lower than it should be?
Have you ever done something that you know just wasn't right? Inside it makes you feel guilty or unhappy, and basically if you can you try to put it right immediately your self-esteem will rocket. Have you heard the words of the song "What have you done today to make you feel proud?" That should be your daily goal to be proud of something you have done every day.

Give yourself permission to nurture yourself.
Praise yourself at every opportunity (usually under your breath), but it's also nice to tell someone how good you felt when you carried something out in an excellent way.

Giving yourself time alone without feeling guilty--saying to the family that you deserve this time and they should respect it-- will help you to learn to enjoy your own company.

SELF ESTEEM

# STAR OF LIFE

Brian Tracy is one of America's leading authorities on the development of human potential and the enhancement of personal effectiveness.

Tracy's programme *"The Psychology of Selling"* suggests standing in front of a mirror and saying to yourself "I like myself, I like myself" several times in a row but I like the idea of praising something you have done while looking in the mirror.
I'll give you an example.

Diane worked with older people in a care home and she could see that Jessie Elder, a client in the home was getting quite agitated. She managed to find out that Jessie was gradually losing her sight and she was becoming totally overwhelmed by her disability. Diane got in touch with the Royal National Institute for the Blind and managed to organise a meeting with another elderly lady who had coped well with her blindness.

Gradually, Jessie, with the help of her new friend, calmed down and started to learn about the things she could still do despite her worsening blindness. That evening when Diane was standing in front of the mirror, she praised herself and just enjoyed those feelings inside knowing she had helped someone. Diane's self-esteem was on the rise.

Is there something tangible which is making you think less of yourself?
For some people it's when they start communicating to someone that they feel inadequate. This is where you have to start improving your vocabulary.

You can easily learn a new word from the dictionary every day--that's 365 in a year! Imagine what that would do for your communication skills.

You may be feeling uncomfortable about your body and that is lowering your self-esteem. Read about Clodagh's success in the Star of Life section on exercise and diet to alter your score upwards.

It's the same as everything else-- what do you want? Where on the scale should you be? Why are you not there and then develop a bite size plan?

# STAR OF LIFE

## STRESS

Now let's look at stress on the Star of Life. Where have you put your cross on that scale if you choose 0% as being the ultimate in unhealthy stress-- and I'll talk about the meaning of healthy and unhealthy stress shortly-- and 100% as being relaxed and balanced in life?

The meaning of "stress" in the Concise Oxford Dictionary is *"a constraining or compelling force,"* and you can imagine something pulling you or crushing you depending whether it is constructive or destructive in your life.

When we all used to live in caves, the "fear, fight and flight" system in our bodies to deal with stress when our lives were in danger, was an essential part of our survival.

Our bodies are given a huge boost of the hormone noradrenaline, which allows us to run with almost super- human speed or gives us extra strength. We have all heard stories of the mother who finding her child trapped beneath a lorry used super human strength to lift the heavy weight. When she returned to the scene later and tried to lift the truck again, she found it impossible! These "stress" hormones are released all the time in our modern lives-- driving cars, dealing with difficult customers, work colleagues, bosses, family members, bereavement and illness.

Our blood pressures rise, our breathing becomes shallower and faster, we sometimes sweat and our bodies divert the blood supply from the digestive organs to our muscles.

Do you remember at school at the start of a race when your gut felt as if it was full of butterflies as you prepared to react to the starting gun?

On the other hand, we need a certain amount of stress to live and we probably wouldn't achieve very much or accomplish most of the advances in civilization without it. So "good" stress is important for getting things done. It is only when stress becomes chronic that it starts to become bad for you.

STRESS

# STAR OF LIFE

What do we normally do with all these "bad stress" hormones flooding our bodies? Probably nothing. Instead of doing some aerobic exercise we usually flop in front of the television after retelling the whole catastrophic detail of how stressed we felt today, which of course just adds to the already damaging effect of unhealthy stress in our bodies. This prolonged state of "activated stress response" can make you ill, and accelerates ageing.

How can we "de-stress" our lives so that we minimise the chronic stress? The first thing you have to do is identify the things in your life that are causing unhealthy stress.

Be honest and write out those things that you know are adversely affecting you. I'll give you a couple of examples of stress that was identified by two people that tried out the life plan, Star of Life.

The first was a lady, Kathleen who in her 50's had to deal with her elderly father who had become quite cantankerous in his old age.

He had such a vicious tongue that it made her ill trying to cope with all his relentless daily jibes. She had marked herself as 10% of a de-stressed life so things were obviously getting on top of her.

As with all the other points on the star, Kathleen had to write down what it was she desired. She wanted to be able to visit her father without becoming upset. I thought the last point was quite significant, since, the only person that can affect how she feels about a situation is Kathleen herself.

She didn't need to write down very much to stimulate her thoughts on how good it would be to be de-stressed and what was going to happen if she continued coping with this level of stress.

Kathleen's main problem was that she didn't feel in control of the situation so she had to work on her association with the unpleasant experience and try and disassociate that feeling when she visited her father.

# STAR OF LIFE

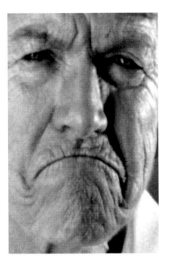

Neuro-Linguistic Programming looks at these concepts and suggests by changing *how* you think you can transform *what* you think. When her father shouted at her, what was she feeling inside? She said she felt like a small child again, as if she was being punished. The disassociation technique I'm about to describe meant that Kathleen was able to play the part of an observer.

Sitting comfortably with her eyes closed she began to imagine what it was like when she was with her father and noted the feelings. She then imagined a pleasant feeling in her life and became fully associated-- stepping inside herself, looking out experiencing those sights and sounds.

To disassociate herself from the feelings she experienced with her father, she imagined the exchange between herself and her father was as if she was watching a movie, totally remote from herself. She then associated the pleasant feelings to watching the movie and she did this pattern several times until it seemed automatic. When she went back to visit her father, she "disassociated" herself from his comments and was able to cope with his jibes. The fact that she was back in control of her feelings meant her stress levels dropped markedly.

The other example is a young man, Gavin, who in his early thirties finds himself really stressed both with his home life (married with a new baby) and work where unless you come in earlier and leave later than everyone else, you are regarded as dispensable. His score on the Star of Life was just 20% of his ideal.

I'm sure you know what had to happen first. Yes, he wrote down what sort of life he wanted in order to create the balance he needed to reduce stress. He then wrote out all the great things that would happen when this unhealthy stress was reduced.

On the next page he noted all the things that might happen if he didn't sort out these problems. One of the first things he wrote down on this page was the affect this constant stress was having on his health.

# STAR OF LIFE

He was developing almost a daily headache and his sleep pattern was unpredictable. Therefore, to continue without change was going to lead to a serious health problem. This gave him all the reason he needed for changing his life.

One of the stressful situations he experienced when he got back from work each day was that he found his wife Eileen, tired and irritable and also a little jealous of the fact that he had been meeting people.

Eileen had decided to give up her own managerial position when the baby was due and felt that she was making a huge sacrifice. Part of the stress in Gavin's life was the effect Eileen was having on him.

He complained that it was all very well to say that his feelings were his own responsibility but because he loved his wife and son he had to solve this quickly before he began to resent the people who were most important to him.

So how do you stop someone else affecting you? In this case, we decided to involve Eileen in the process to find out what she wanted as well as Gavin.

As expected, she wanted Gavin to show he valued her and their new baby by spending more time at home. Eileen also wanted to be able to go out sometimes without her child, so Gavin had to examine his work schedule. With the sort of work he undertook it was possible to be flexible in terms of time spent at the office.

Gavin developed a plan involving a work schedule that meant he was home one hour earlier every night. He could also afford to take a half-day off per month by working "smarter" rather than "harder".

With any plan from the Star of Life, you have to *do* something right away to start the momentum, so he telephoned his boss's secretary to ask for an appointment. This was scheduled for the following week, and when the day arrived he had carefully prepared his case making sure that his boss fully understood that all the work would be done but that Gavin's time schedule would have to be agreed.

# STAR OF LIFE

When his boss saw how much effort Gavin had put into his argument, he readily agreed with the new arrangement and announced what was happening to all the other staff.

Gavin came home earlier every night and this meant he could help Eileen with the baby.

The half-day off he had negotiated was written in his diary as a "special" afternoon with his family. In other words, if anyone asked him to take part in something that afternoon, he would look up his diary and say,

"I'm sorry, I've already got an appointment".

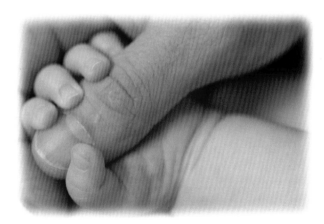

Gavin also made sure that Eileen got some time to herself and he made her phone a girlfriend to set a weekly date--every Thursday evening--to do some exercise together at the local gym or just go out for a drink or a meal.

By making sure his wife was happy, the stress he was feeling virtually disappeared.

And guess what? Their relationship soared.

# STAR OF LIFE

I hope these examples of how to deal with "bad" stress will give you ideas to help you experience the sort of life you deserve. What is your level on the chart? Then decide where you want to be and devise a plan to get there. Of course the most important part of your plan is to take action today

So let's finish with some general points on reducing stress:

You need to accept what you can't control by altering your attitude to it.
Try some "disassociation" techniques, then take some action.

You probably spend a lot of time worrying about things that will never happen.
Do an experiment. Write down everything you are worrying about today and one month later check to see what actually happened. You will find that the vast majority of what you worried about is totally irrelevant.

If you feel overwhelmed by what you have to do then make a list. Try and prioritise the list according to the importance of the task, for example if you were asked to go on an assignment abroad for one month what are the things you must do before you leave? What are the things that would be nice to do before you leave but are not a must and how about the items that really aren't that important? Once your list is more manageable start your important items today.

Take some time out every day to help your mind and body recover. Every hour, can you close your eyes for a few seconds? To rest your eyes-- particularly if you've been working on a computer-- rub your hands together to generate heat and then, with cupped hands, place them over your closed eyes for as long as you can. This will rest your eyes and help de-stress your mind.

For your body, there is an example in the **Alexander Technique**
set of exercises to help with stress.

# STAR OF LIFE

I like to de-stress by using a position loosely based on this technique.

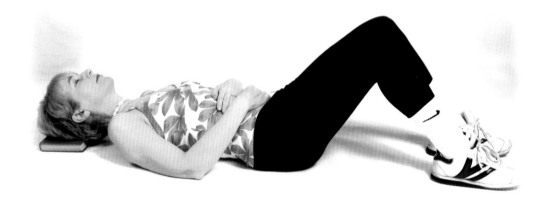

Frederick Matthias devised the Alexander Technique as a way of learning how to "co-operate" with the mechanism nature has given us to support ourselves against gravity.

I first came across the concept some years ago after I was involved in a car accident. (Someone ran into the back of my car at speed while I was stationary at traffic lights.)

I suffered a whiplash injury involving my neck and back and despite intensive physiotherapy I was left with a great deal of pain. After ten lessons from a practitioner the pain ceased and I was able to resume my normal movement including sport.

Please ensure that you take advice from a qualified Alexander Technique practitioner before attempting any positions.

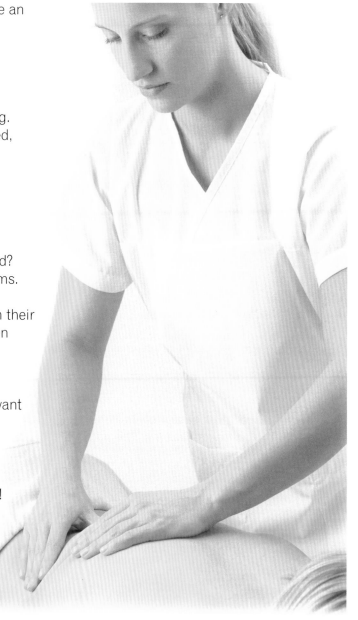

# STAR OF LIFE

Another way to de-stress your body is to have an aromatherapy massage.

Book yourself in once a week and just enjoy the experience.

Look at the section on oxygen about laughing. If you can't laugh because you're too stressed, try at least smiling. Smiling will release endorphins in the brain and that will make you feel more relaxed.

Change the word "problems" to "opportunities". Can you imagine someone (hopefully not you) frowning with head bowed? That person is obviously dealing with problems.

Lets turn it around and look at someone with their head up--excited, looking for inspiration-- then that person is dealing with opportunities. Guess who is less stressed?

If you've planned the things you absolutely want to do then you should be less stressed.

Look at life as if it is a wonderful gift.

You don't have time to have any "bad" stress!

# STAR OF LIFE

## CAREER

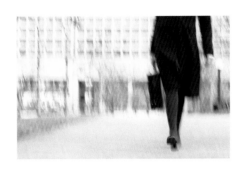

Check out your percentage as far as work and career is concerned--0% means you don't have a job and would like one and 100% is where you're flying high and living your dream job.

Say you're in a job that you really don't like. You're probably about 30% of your potential on the Star of Life grid.

The first thing to do before abandoning where you are is to look at the factors concerning your unrest. If it's the boss, then is it how he or she is treating you? What about recognition for what you've done?

Have you tried telling your boss how you feel because sometimes the problem can be easily remedied if you confront the person?

The same with work colleagues, if you take the person aside and "have a chat" about what you think is wrong, remember to listen carefully to their point of view before explaining your side, it's incredible how things can be easily sorted. Are you also doing what you're good at and enjoy doing?

CAREER

It's amazing how people can be stuck in a rut at work yet when they are given the extra responsibility or a slight change in direction, they just blossom.

Diane came up with an idea at work for making one of the procedures more efficient. She knew that this change, if implemented, would save the company a great deal of money so she approached her boss.

The company decided to try out her idea, and because it did save money Diane was awarded a pay rise for her efforts. Suddenly her job became much more satisfying.

Find out if there are factors in your job than can be changed before thinking about a move.

# STAR OF LIFE

Let's look at another scenario regarding your career.
What would really appeal to you? Do you have to go to night school, read books, attend seminars or seek out a mentor to help in your quest? If you're serious you will attain the necessary skills in your own time and then you can start the interview process with an eye toward the position you want.

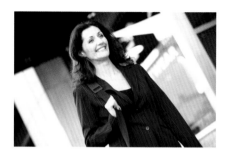

Angela always wanted to work in the design business so she found a distance-learning course that was grant-aided. She had to work at nights and weekends until she got her qualification. Angela didn't mind sacrificing her free time because she knew exactly what she wanted and how to get there.

So how do you think she sounded when she went for interviews?
Of course she was positive, enthusiastic and had the confidence to admit that she had little experience on the topic but was determined to learn quickly from her knowledge base. Employers were only too keen to offer her a position on a trial basis, and Angela knew if she wanted to stay she had to prove herself.

For the self-employed the question I would like to ask is one I heard from Brian Tracy: "If you knew what you know now would you get into that business?" The Star of Life percentage may be as low as 20%. If the answer is "no" then you need to start planning your exit. Is there someone out there that might want to run your business differently and sees good potential?

John ran a successful printing firm but realised that it would be better to be part of a bigger organisation. He started to ask around and eventually was able to strike a deal as a partnership. This meant he was able to step back from the day-to-day running of the business and eventually sold his share when he was ready to move on.

Another example was Andrew who had a small newsagent shop. He found a young couple that wanted to buy into the business as a going concern and he negotiated a deal where the couple took over the business but he still owned the property.

# STAR OF LIFE

Andrew was able to pursue the thing he really wanted to do, which was to play the trumpet in a band while being supported by this small steady income. It's just so gratifying to see someone grow and develop and, in Andrew's case, doing what he loves.

What if you haven't got a job but would love one? (This is where you have a zero percentage on the Star of Life scale.) Notice I use the word "love" because that enthusiasm has to come across to the prospective employer.

What is your attitude to work when you go for an interview? If you never get any interviews and therefore can't demonstrate your enthusiasm then you're not giving the prospective employer what is required in your application.

I'll give you an example of success by describing David, who was out of work but knew he had a wonderful talent for organising people and events. The first thing he needed to do was to look at all the newspaper adverts for companies that could be organising events for promotion but whose owners were too involved in producing the product.

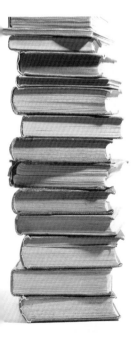

Many companies under perform because they don't market their excellent product. He then needed to look at companies that were doing fantastic promotions and whose shares and profits were booming. All David had to do was to spend some time marrying the ideas to the companies that he felt needed the service and then market the value of the service.

David produced a list of all the compelling benefits the company would derive from his promotion ideas and how David would organise the events. (He had to do a lot of homework to make sure his ideas would produce the kind of return the company was seeking.)

With an abundance of enthusiasm, and self-belief, David set off to visit the companies he had identified would be receptive to his ideas. The first few businesses were not interested. Some were downright rude, whereas others were sceptical.

# STAR OF LIFE

Many people would have given up. David, on the other hand, had been reading some self-development books about how to turn "failure" into opportunity. Instead of feeling downhearted he set about learning all he could from each rejection.

Eventually, his persistence paid off and a small but thriving company liked the idea of David's promotions and signed him up. The next time he plotted his chart he was pushing 60%-- not so much an improvement more a transformation.

You see what the important elements are in David's success story:

- **David believed in himself and in his talent**

- **He worked at finding out the markets that would be interested in his ideas; he targeted his audience**

- **He "sold" his ideas not on what he wanted but on how the companies benefit from taking his service on board.**

As you probably guessed, David exceeded the company's expectations in terms of attracting extra sales and soon other companies wanted him to look at their promotions. It was such an exciting time for David, and if this example relates to you then:

- **Believe in yourself**

- **Ask yourself what benefits the prospective employer should expect from hiring you and then sell your ideas at the interview**

- **If you fail at first, pick yourself up, learn from it and carry on.**

By plotting your present work status on the grid and then projecting that number to where you would like to be, you can propel yourself forward using the ideas in this section and watch your percentage soar! How does that affect the rest of your life when you're working at something you enjoy?

# STAR OF LIFE

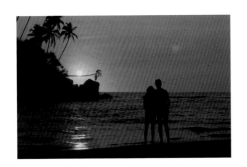

## GOALS

If we pick another topic from the Star--goal setting-- and if we say that once a year you set goals, probably at New Year, and you never write them down, then you're likely to be at about 10% of your potential.

Interestingly, only about 1% of the population have written goals and many don't have any plans to attain them. If you have children, then one of the most useful examples you can give them is to set goals yourself and to encourage them to do the same and watch them stretch and accomplish things that they themselves didn't think possible.

I like to encourage people to write down impossible goals. By that I mean you dream of what you want--not what you think you can attain-- in as much detail as you can and, as you write down these goals (in the present tense as if you have them already accomplished), you need to think of the reasons why you want them.

Thomas Edison, the inventor, was purported to, when writing his goal of developing the electric light bulb, begin envisaging what his invention would do for people.

Can you imagine how much emotion would be associated with the development of such an invention? He wrote down how it would change the world and how much it would help people as well as fulfilling his own personal dream.

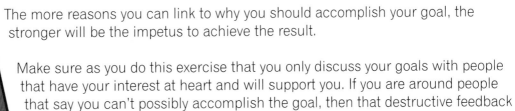

The more reasons you can link to why you should accomplish your goal, the stronger will be the impetus to achieve the result.

Make sure as you do this exercise that you only discuss your goals with people that have your interest at heart and will support you. If you are around people that say you can't possibly accomplish the goal, then that destructive feedback can completely derail your plans.

GOALS

# STAR OF LIFE

That fear of criticism conveyed to us by our peers is such a strong demotivator that it can stop you from ever setting goals in the future.

Also, don't worry about failure. Use it as a learning experience--why did that happen and what can you change to get you back on track?

You need to review your major goals every day preferably, first thing in the morning when your mind is fresh and receptive to ideas.

It may be that the goal you first thought of is actually redundant or needs to be put in another context. It is more important that your goal is still relevant and still fills you with passion and excitement than concern about changing direction.

You also need a coach to make sure you follow through on your goals and to help you make the journey much easier.

Be at 80-90% of your goal achievement on the Star of Life and feel fantastic.

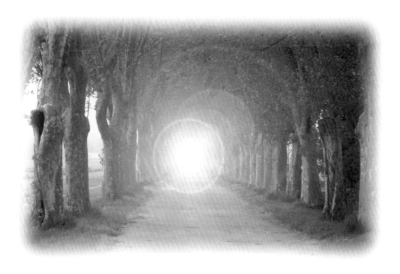

# STAR OF LIFE

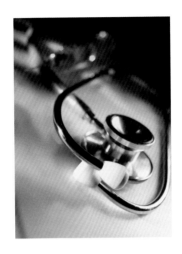

## HEALTH

Where do you rate yourself in terms of health? Remember that good health isn't just the absence of disease but feeling fully energised most of the time.

To help you decide what your percentage is on the scale, refer to the "Markers of our Biological Age" and book yourself in for an "MOT" for health.

What do I mean by an MOT? Well, a lot of doctor practices run "well-man or-woman" clinics where an assessment is done using standard tests. Some pharmacies as well can check your blood in terms of cholesterol or blood glucose and have facilities for measuring your blood pressure and body mass index. *(See below for explanation.)*

The cholesterol test can tell you if your blood is healthy in terms of fat content. You have "good" cholesterol and "bad" cholesterol values in the test and the practitioner uses those results as well as blood pressure, level of obesity, family history and smoking habits to work out how much risk you have in terms of heart disease.

There are normal measurements for blood pressure according to your age, and your blood test for "sugar" in the blood will let you know if there is a risk of diabetes.

Body mass index is just a fancy expression for one of the assessments for obesity using your height and weight. The MOT test uses your weight in kilograms, divided by your height in metres, squared.

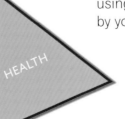

$$BMI = \frac{\textbf{weight} \text{ (kgs)}}{\textbf{height} \text{ (metres) squared}}$$

If that number is more than 25 then you need to lose weight.

# STAR OF LIFE

Once these measurements are taken your health professional can explain where you are in terms of health and how you can improve things using lifestyle indicators.

Maybe you would like to give them a copy of the book since you can show them how you are going to improve your health using the 10 steps.

But what about the other markers for your "Biological Age"?
How do you get them assessed?

Some private clinics do all the tests listed, and there are sports clinics that will check your aerobic capacity *(see section on oxygen)*.

Bone density is a measurement looking at your risk of osteoporosis or whether you are likely to break bones with a simple fall.

Although there are tests in some clinics, the gold standard is something called a **"dexa scan"** which measures bone density for people considered to be at risk of breaking bones.

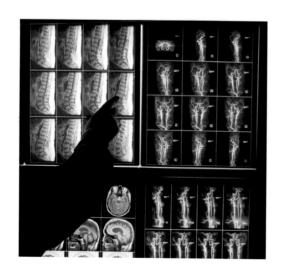

# STAR OF LIFE

One interesting blood test that can give you information about your underlying health such as nutritional deficiencies and the state of your liver is called "**Live Blood Microscopy**".

Only one drop of blood is required (from a pin-prick to the fingertip) and this is viewed on a monitor. *(Details of availability on information page)*

With all those tests you may find that you have to do a little bit of work to get yourself back into shape, but the good thing is you have all the steps to get you there –just refer to the relevant chapter.

As I stated at the beginning of this section, how you feel each day is a true measure of your health status.

Where are you on the scale and how do you want to feel because you can change things if you want to?

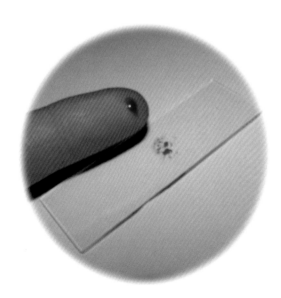

# STAR OF LIFE

Deborah went to a private clinic to get all the tests done and found, as she suspected, she was healthy but unfit.

She put her mark on the 60% health line but only 20% on the exercise line since the only exercise she did was some walking at lunchtime.

Because she seriously wanted to get fit, she started doing 15 minutes of "power walking" every day.

This is where you walk briskly swinging your arms and focussing on expending a reasonable amount of energy as you move.

Rebounding was another exercise she started and spent 10 minutes rebounding and listening to her favourite music. In the evening she exercised using the Swiss Ball *(see chapter 5)*.

She felt better as she increased her aerobic capacity
*(see section on oxygen)*.

That of course is the key to having an enjoyable life-- you have to feel brilliant most of the time.

Deborah achieved a marvellous result when she returned after six months for a re-test and found her "Biological Age" had gone down by five years.

Her percentage on the Star of Life scale had risen to 80%. Yes, you can do the same!

# STAR OF LIFE

## DIET & FITNESS

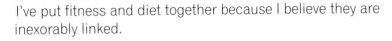

I've put fitness and diet together because I believe they are inexorably linked.

Apart from suggesting you look at the chapters on exercise and diet, I thought I would illustrate how the Star of Life worked for an Irish lady called Clodagh.

On the fitness scale, Clodagh admitted she was 10% of what she should be. She didn't exercise at all and her work involved sitting in an office for most of her day.

We started with looking at the reasons she wanted to exercise and it was very much the usual motives of improving health, reducing weight and generally wanting to be happier about her appearance.

The desire for change needs to be much stronger than that so we started to delve deep into what the consequences of **not exercising** were and also the benefits of starting. That's what you have to do to get yourself motivated to do something that, at first, seems quite painful.

Clodagh got herself hyped up with her reasons for starting the programme. She was truly determined to carry it through. This determination is critical to success.

Make sure you get yourself to that level before you start by writing out all the factors that need to be taken into account to motivate you.

DIET

Clodagh looked at what she liked to do and the first activity on the list was walking, so with appropriate questioning we devised an exercise programme with walking at the core.

# STAR OF LIFE

Then Clodagh managed to identify a friend, Irene, who, equally determined, would make sure that she performed her twenty minutes of brisk walking every day. Clodagh could easily walk to work but we both felt that with the possible bad weather, arriving at work soaked to the skin, might not be the best start to the day and that might put her off.

I also discovered that she used to enjoy swimming but now felt embarrassed about her figure. Nevertheless she scheduled a half-hour swim once a week with the idea to increase to twice a week after one month. It was relatively easy to find a pool that had a club for middle aged swimmers and beyond who had such a range of body sizes and shapes that Clodagh easily blended in.

With an aim toward being stronger and having better balance Clodagh bought herself a rebounder. *(See section on exercise.)*

Ten minutes of rebounding was fitted into her routine before breakfast. This meant she had to set her alarm 15 minutes earlier in the morning but that wasn't a problem for her.

Clodagh loved to watch television so we worked through a series of exercises to improve the strength of her arms and legs while sitting. For her legs, sitting on a table with her legs dangling she hung a pot of paint over her foot and tried to lift her leg up (each one in turn).

It was incredibly difficult at first, but over the next 10 days she managed to lift each leg to a horizontal level holding the position for 5 seconds at a time.

For her arms she used two pots of jam *(see illustrations in exercise section)* and was happy to carry out the exercises while watching her favourite TV programmes.

The feeling of achievement kept Clodagh going. She was able to plot her improvement on the Star of Life grid that gave her the impetus to get to the next level.

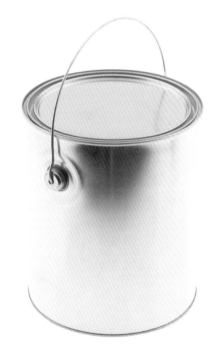

# STAR OF LIFE

She and her friend Irene cajoled each other into carrying on with the plan.

Have you got a friend that is looking to get fit as well?

Research has shown that if you regularly exercise for six months then you will always exercise since your body will ultimately miss the activity if you give up.

Clodagh was overweight, so before she embarked on her programme she checked herself into the doctor's surgery for advice on the appropriateness of the regime.

Her doctor looked at the prepared schedule and sanctioned the exercises with the proviso that she should stop immediately if she did feel uncomfortable.

As I said at the beginning of this section, exercise and diet are inexorably linked to losing weight since you have to move as well as eat a nutritious diet to get results.

The diet side proved to be an easier option since Clodagh's daughter was getting married in six months.

It was a fantastic incentive since in one of those mad moments that only women seem to have, she had bought herself the "mother-of-the-bride' outfit of her dreams. The only problem was that it was a size 14. At least two sizes less than at present.

Once we made sure that the incentive was firmly embedded --since after all she would have nothing to wear come the wedding--Clodagh then visualised herself looking pretty spectacular in her size 14 outfit and experienced the feelings of achievement she would get when following through on her plan.

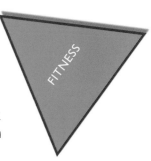

The visualisation and imagination step of how you are likely to look and feel when you master your goal are keys to your success when making difficult changes.

# STAR OF LIFE

These were the steps to Clodagh's new eating habits:

1. The refrigerator was raided and all unsuitable produce was given away or thrown out.

2. She then made a list of all the new alkalising foods *(see section on diet)* that she would need to have including a lot of food that she would enjoy.

3. A daily chart was created containing very filling, tasty dishes with ideas for nutritious snacks.

4. Irene and herself had a weekly weigh-in and measurement on a Friday night and, provided that they had both been disciplined in terms of eating and exercise, they then went for their treat.

   They both loved ice cream, so their treat was to have a double scoop with chocolate sauce. The interesting thing was that, previously they would have been tempted to have a second helping but now because of the change of diet both of them were satisfied with the one helping.

5. To increase her metabolic rate, Clodagh spent a few minutes on her rebounder before her evening meal.

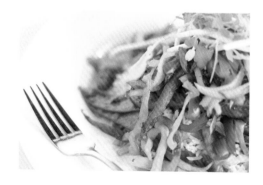

# STAR OF LIFE

The importance of Clodagh's success was that it was a lasting change.

There would be no point in her fitting the size 14 outfit at the wedding and then returning to the old ways immediately afterwards.

Clodagh had trained her body to sustain her fitness and eating habits well beyond the wedding day.

I must tell you about her daughter's wedding.
Clodagh had a wonderful time. She looked and felt like a million dollars, dancing every dance without feeling tired and accepting all the compliments that were showered upon her by people that were amazed at her transformation.

Long after the event, the wedding photographs were a constant reminder of her achievement and gave her the incentive never to return to the way she was before.

Remember the Star of Life is not a quick fix. It's an approach to lasting change.

# STAR OF LIFE

As far as my own life, I plotted where I was, percentage-wise, about three years ago and developed an illustration that reflected my imbalance. I got a blood test taken when I was going through a cleansing and rejuvenating week in Fiji whilst on the Anthony Robbins Mastery University course.

That blood test reflected the stress I was under, the acidity of my blood and the disparity between my mineral levels and those of a healthy individual. These results bore out the fact that I had to change in almost every area of my life if I wanted to feel energised, alive and improve my overall health.

Upon returning from my trip, I immediately started to change virtually every aspect of my life. I had always said that, although my day job involves standing maybe for nine hours, standing doesn't actually reflect quality exercise. I bought myself a rebounder and started a 10-minute programme to build up my muscles, help prevent osteoporosis and give me energy to start my day.

I take time to meditate and have some quiet reflection first thing in the morning and then I do a brisk walk outside for 15 minutes with incantations, 10 deep breaths (see section on oxygen) then stretching exercises using the sun salutation yoga postures.

Some strength exercises such as press-ups are performed in the middle of my morning routine while others such as thigh exercises are usually completed in the evening with the Swiss Ball.

My liquid colloidal minerals are taken first thing along with a small measure (30ml) of Noni juice. Noni juice is derived from the noni plant grown mainly in Tahiti and Hawaii. Its properties suggest it has a healing effect and, although I think I am reasonably healthy I have decided to include the drink in my morning regime as an insurance measure.

After my exercise, I take fruit and an essential fatty acid oil blend. My breakfast consists of a salad/vegetable mix with humous and organic porridge oats with flaxseed.

# STAR OF LIFE

I take my powerful antioxidant supplements both after breakfast and in the evening. The 1.7litres of filtered water I drink daily includes 200ml first thing and drinking the rest in between meals throughout the day and into the evening. I have a reverse osmosis water filter fitted at home. *(information about this can be found at the back of the book.)*

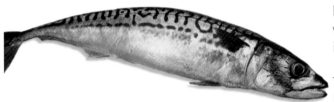

I eat a lot of oily fish, salads and vegetables and my treat every so often is a small cappuccino with a piece of chocolate.

This all means that my diet, fitness and, ultimately, health are all standing at a very high percentage and I feel like a different person.

When I looked at my finances I decided to write down exactly what I wanted to earn this year. I knew if I worked at certain aspects of my financial plan, wrote down the reasons for earning that amount and the consequences of not doing so, things should start to happen. This is exactly what has transpired so, for myself, the Star of Life works.

I knew my high stress levels were mainly caused by my work. I have since systematically delegated more of my duties to others as well as taking more time out to either enjoy a holiday or pursue the areas of interest relating to my business.

I find that the quality of my sleep has improved. I actually need less sleep because, I presume, my body and mind are being nourished by reducing the daily stress and my body is being given the tools I need with the nutritious food and supplements I ingest on a daily basis.

In addition I was not spending enough time with my husband and so I have altered my activities to make sure that some of our outside interests involve both of us. In general, I try to constantly grow and learn and attend many courses on self improvement.

# STAR OF LIFE

Anthony Robbins runs a programme called *"Date With Destiny"* and one of the tasks you are assigned is to compose a mission statement for your life. This examines the purpose of your life and determines what you really like to do.

You need to imagine a time when something you did was effortless. Another person might find that task so difficult yet you made it look easy.

You are now starting to discover what you must do with your life to bring you fulfilment. You need to look at your values and rules both from the point of view of moving towards your purpose in life and also those rules and values that take you in the opposite direction.

Say your main purpose was to be happy and with that happiness you can offer to make other people happy. Your "for" rules and values may include whenever you smile or laugh or appreciate someone else's happiness you are moving towards your mission statement.

Those against, or "moving away from" rules and values, could include unhappiness reflected in not smiling or laughing every day. Just sit and dream about why you are here, then start to build up values and rules that propel you to where you want to go.

For myself, I know my purpose is to help as many people as possible to feel better-- which is probably why I wrote this book. I have personally found such a difference in my energy levels and my outlook on life that I need to share this widely.

Look at the following steps implement as much as you can and improve the quality of your life, and remember to have fun!

**You can find more information and download printable copies of The Star of Life--Life Plan on the website**

www.newlifehealthcare.co.uk

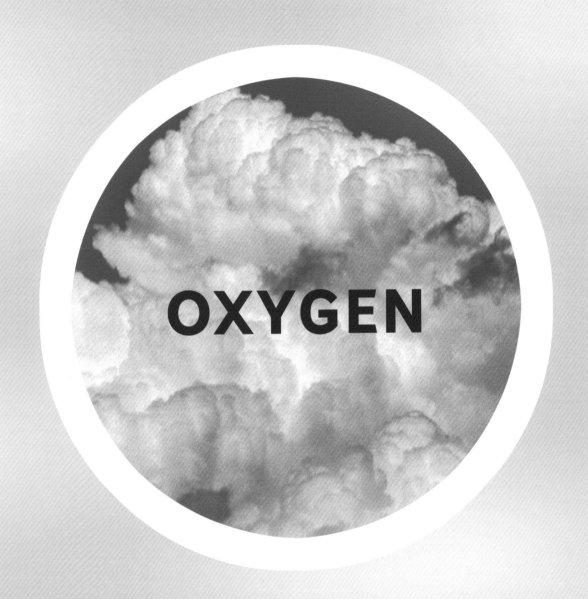

OXYGEN

"So long as men can breathe,
or eyes can see,
so long lives this,
and this gives life to thee"

**Shakespeare (Sonnet 18**)

# OXYGEN

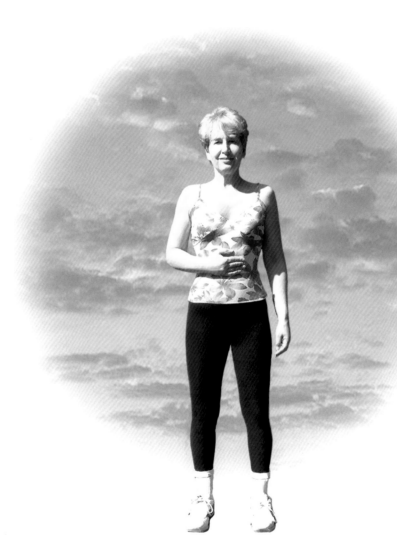

Stand up, I want you to experience the benefit of increased oxygen intake.

Stand with your feet, shoulder width apart, and put the palm of your hand on your diaphragm.
*(This is located just below the rib cage.)*

I now want you to take a large intake of breath through the nostrils for a count of two, hold your breath for a count of eight and then exhale steadily through the mouth for a count of four.

You should feel your stomach moving out when you breathe in and the opposite as you breathe out.

Most people, when you ask them to take a deep breath, raise their shoulders as an automatic reflex.

Trained singers and actors know that, to gain optimum performance, they need to breathe from the diaphragm.

The shoulders should stay largely fixed and it's your stomach that moves in and out as you breathe.

# OXYGEN

Many of us go through our lives not breathing correctly and thus depriving the body of its full supply of oxygen.

Shallow breathing decreases the body's ability to eliminate carbon dioxide more thoroughly. The tissues have less oxygen from the blood pumped through the body and waste material is less capable of being eliminated via the lymphatic system.

No wonder we feel lacking in energy at times during the day that in turn can have a detrimental effect on our emotional well-being.

Try this form of breathing 10 times at least once a day, particularly first thing in the morning to really give your energy levels a boost.

Oxygen is an essential element required for our body to properly function.
When inhaled it is transported by blood to all parts of the body, combining with haemoglobin in the red blood cells.

Dietary nutrients, such as carbohydrates, fats and proteins require oxygen to convert our food to energy.

How vital is sufficient oxygen to the human body? Well, many experts believe that lack of oxygen in human cells and tissue is linked to a vast variety of health problems and diseases.

Dr. Otto Warburg, twice Nobel laureate, stated that "the primary cause of cancer is the replacement of normal oxygen respiration of body cells by anaerobic (oxygen-deficient) cell respiration." In other words, cancer cells thrive in a medium with little oxygen.

So how do we feel when we are oxygen deficient? Well, as you would expect, there is an overall weakness, fatigue and poor circulation.

Lack of oxygen can compromise the immune system. That means that the body is more susceptible to viruses and infections.

# OXYGEN

Apart from the breathing exercise what else can we do to increase our oxygen intake?

Aerobic exercise, for example, means the body is utilising oxygen efficiently through increasing the blood supply to the tissues.

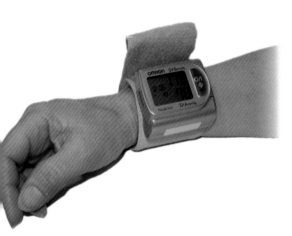

Use a wrist pulse metre to work out your aerobic heart rate by subtracting your age from 220.
*(for obtaining your own pulse meter see information page).*

If you are able to increase your pulse to 75-85% of this figure for 20 minutes, three times a week, then you will find that your level of fitness will improve dramatically.

Remember to warm up and cool down as well for five minutes either end of the exercise.

To be sure, if you are consulting a doctor for a medical condition, then you need to find out the appropriate type of exercise before starting.

You need to enjoy exercise whether it's team games or dancing to your favourite music.

*(See the section on exercise for some ideas).*

# OXYGEN

One simple way to increase oxygen intake is to laugh.
Do you remember laughing so much as a child at the breakfast table
that the milk from the cereal came down your nose?

As Josh Billings, the American humorist said

> *"Laughing is the sensation of feeling good all over
> and showing it principally in one spot."*

There are a lot of physiological benefits from laughing.
There is an increased consumption of oxygen as well as an increase
in the heart and respiratory rate.

The serum level of the stress hormone decreases and the immune system
is stimulated.

The muscles of the face and stomach have a real workout and in fact,
I have heard laughing referred to as "internal jogging"!

Norman Cousins, author of "Anatomy of an Illness" suffered from insomnia
due to severe inflammation of the spine and joints.

He used to prescribe himself bellyaching laughter
from videos in order to promote pain-free sleep.

A team of psychologists at Glasgow Caledonian University
used comedian Billy Connolly's recordings to find
alternatives to anaesthetics.

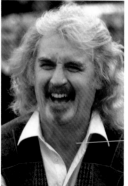

They found that men in the experiments were able to
tolerate their hands in freezing water for three times
as long while listening to Connolly's comedy routines.

# OXYGEN

Another simple way of taking more oxygen into the body is by singing loudly and with great force. Edwin Coppard in his book "Sovereign Singing" teaches people to sing using his knowledge of human physiology and music:

- Sit up straight, open your mouth and start to sing a note out as loudly as possible. Do this while swaying your body back and forward.

- Imagine you are singing each note on a scale but with great gusto.

- Sing ah, ah, ah, ah all at the same tone then change up a little and continue with the ah, ahs right up the scale before going back down to the original note.

- Try a sequence of notes still at the same intensity and listen to your voice. Yes, you have a reasonable voice and I bet you feel energised!

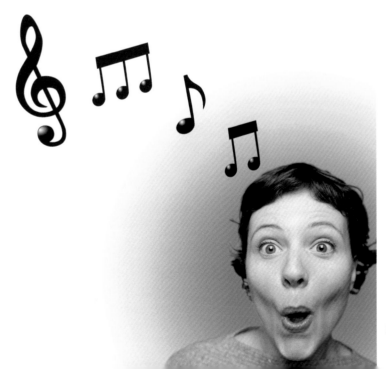

# OXYGEN

The benefits of getting the right amount of oxygen into the body can be both physically and mentally stimulating as shown below.

- **Re-energises**

- **Increases alertness**

- **Increases concentration**

- **Reduces tiredness**

- **Promotes relaxation**

- **Promotes healthy looking skin**

- **Reduces the build up of lactic acid following exercise.**

### Step 2 - Get more oxygen into your body

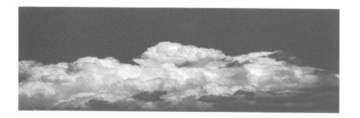

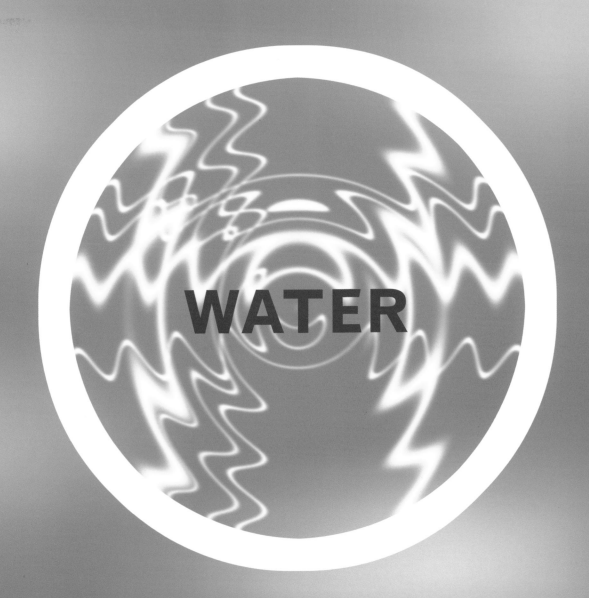

WATER

*"Water is fundamental for life and health"*

**The United Nations Committee on Economic,**

**Cultural and Social Rights.**

# WATER

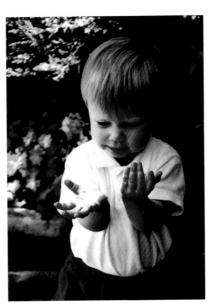

What is it about water that makes us spend our holidays beside it, swim in it, relax and bathe in it, and even experience therapies with it? Are we naturally drawn to water perhaps because water makes up approximately 75% of our bodies?

Water is essential for living and without it we could die in a few days. We don't drink enough water nowadays and we are not always aware we are dehydrated. In fact, feeling "thirsty", is probably the last sensation of dehydration the body experiences. Before that, we sometimes experience lethargy, lack of concentration, and are more vulnerable to stress so, one of the easiest ways of giving yourself more energy is to increase your consumption of water.

So how much water should we drink?

Everyone should drink about 8 to 10 glasses of water per day depending on your weight.

Try calculating your weight in pounds. Remember, 10 stones equal 140 lbs. Then divide your weight by 2 and multiply the result by 30 the approximate number of millilitres in a fluid ounce.

In this example this equals 2.1 litres. The tall bottles of water that we sometimes buy from the supermarket usually contain about 1.5 litres so that gives you an idea of the daily amount you actually need.

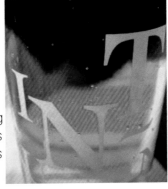

You cannot go from zero water (I'm not talking about teas, coffees or fruit juices) to 1.5 litres of water all in a day. You should look at the different fluids you drink in a day. Gradually start substituting water for coffees, juices and fizzy drinks. Diet drinks are not recommended since they contain impurities the body has to work hard to eliminate.

**69**

# WATER

As you start to drink more water, you will adjust and you will spend less time rushing to the bathroom, as the body will know that it will always receive the right amount of water for its needs.

If you feel worried as to what might happen at the other end when you take more water, then exercises to strengthen the pelvic floor muscles can help. These exercises can't replace expert advice and assessment from a trained continence nurse. (The following example is for women.)

Always sit on the toilet seat as opposed to "drooping" and, in order to locate the right muscles, try to stop the flow of urine midstream. You should do this once only to feel the muscles contracting.

Normally, allow the urine to flow freely and try to empty the bladder a second time after you think you've finished. Never ignore the urge to go to the bathroom because you're too busy.

You must try to perform pelvic floor exercises several times a day if you feel you have a problem. Draw the muscles up inside you for a count of five then relax, releasing slowly. Rest in between each contraction and, after performing approximately 5 slow contractions, finish with another 10, this time releasing quickly. Always remember to breathe evenly throughout.

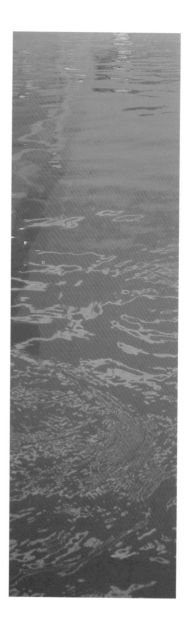

# WATER

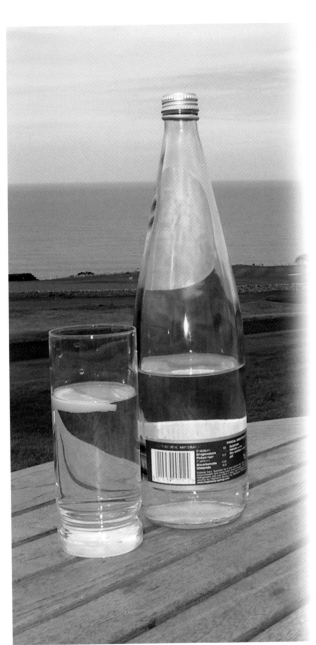

In order to ensure that you drink enough water throughout the day, you need to start first thing in the morning because your body is dehydrated after sleep. Have a mug of water with a slice of lemon. beside your bed and, if you spend your time travelling to work, drink a 250ml (8oz) bottle during that time. During the morning continue to drink a couple of glasses of water, but take your last drink of the morning half an hour before lunch.

Do you want to lose weight? Sometimes when we feel hungry we actually need water. In fact if you take a large glass of water half an hour before food you won't eat as much. Remember water should be at room temperature because it's harder for the body to absorb, the colder it is and ideally, you should sip it continuously rather than gulp it down in large quantities. This gives the body a better chance to absorb the fluid.

Don't drink while you are eating or for half an hour after completion of the meal as this can affect your digestion of food. Carry on drinking water in the afternoon and again stop half an hour before your evening meal. Take the last of the allotted daily amount up to about a couple of hours before bed since you don't want to have your sleep disturbed. This routine may seem quite difficult to manage but, once you start drinking more water, you will actually start to feel thirsty if you drink less.

# WATER

Some danger times for the onset of dehydration are during air travel (some airlines give you glasses of water at regular intervals) hot weather and exercise, when you are most likely to perspire.

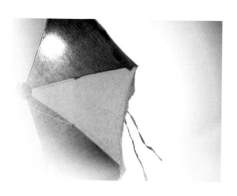

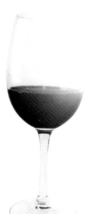

These are times when you should compensate by increasing your water intake. Alcohol, of course, causes dehydration. For every unit of alcohol for example, a glass of wine, the body loses the same amount of water.

That's because water is used in the process of eliminating alcohol from the body.

With so much emphasis on drinking water, how do you decide what type you should drink? I've always felt tap water is best but I would recommend filtering the water first to remove impurities and chemical additives since I feel these have a detrimental effect on the body. As I said earlier, I use a reverse osmosis filtering system.

When you are travelling, it may be necessary to use bottled water but choose one packaged in glass rather than plastic. Chemicals may leach into the contents of the bottle from plastic containers.

While plain water is always the best, if you want to consume flavoured drinks rather than tea, coffee or carbonated beverages you can always try some of the interesting herbal drinks.

**Camomile**
 helps reduce anxiety, headaches and insomnia, as well as soothing the nervous and digestive systems.

**Lemon balm**
 lifts the spirits if you're feeling depressed or suffer from nervous indigestion.

**Peppermint**
 is good for travel sickness, the relief of headaches and as a general pick- me- up.

# WATER

The Iranian-born Dr. Fereydoon Batmanghelidj, has written a book called "Your body's many cries for water" in which he promotes water as curative for many of our western diseases and conditions.

He believes, as I do, that sufficient water combined with a nutritious diet and exercise are the three most vital and basic anti-ageing precautions for good health. When your skin is well hydrated, it looks good and that in turn makes you feel good.

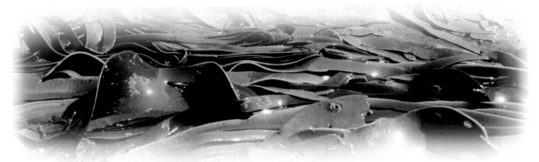

Finally, from the Christian ritual of baptism to swimming and general bathing, water provides a calming and yet uplifting effect on the mind. If you suffer from an injury or have a chronic condition that makes normal exercise difficult or painful, water provides the ideal medium for exercising, using its buoyancy as a protective.

Find out if there is an aqua aerobic class in your area. They are usually designed for a large spectrum of needs from general fitness to antenatal requirements. Meditating near an ocean with the rhythmic sound of moving water stills the mind, giving a sense of tranquillity and, of course, there are the benefits of minerals from the sea absorbed while bathing.

Thallasotherapy is a form of hydrotherapy that uses seawater

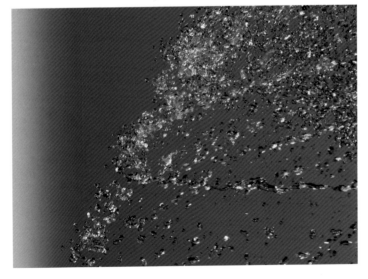

# WATER

or other substances such as mud extracted from the sea as well as sand, seaweed and minerals.

Treat yourself to a body wrap containing rich concentrations of the Dead Sea salts or lie and meditate in a flotation pool. You deserve it.

Some hydrotherapy treatments consist of hot - and cold-water applications. Saunas and steam baths produce sweating which in turn allows both the muscles and the mind to relax. Alternating treatments between hot and cold are believed to build up immunity and can increase vitality.

Water is such an important component of every day life; make sure you make the best use of it. Enjoy the world's valuable resource for energy and well-being.

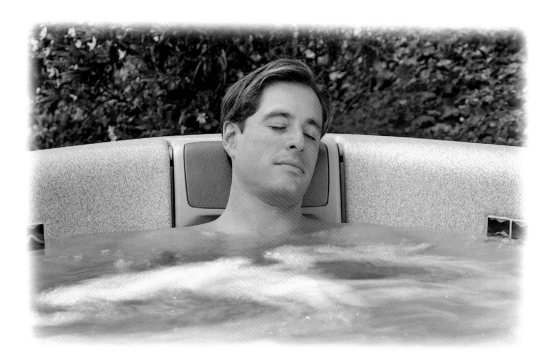

**Step 3 - Enjoy and consume more water on a daily basis**

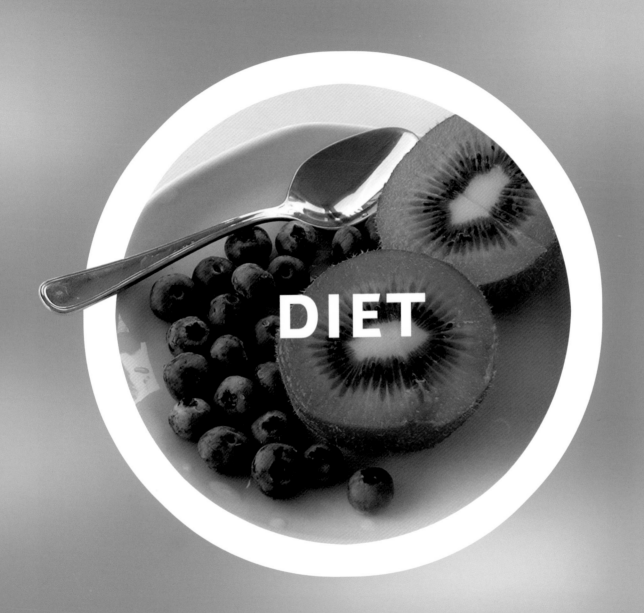

*"Food can be your medicine
and medicine can be your food"*

**Hippocrates**

# DIET

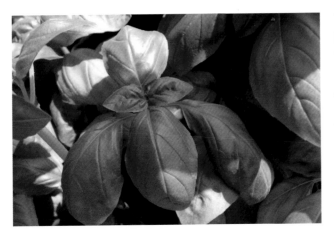

There is no doubt that we are what we eat. Our bodies need the essential building blocks in our food to keep us healthy and energised.

A physical and spiritual transformation takes place when you start to choose the appropriate food for your body.

There are many references relating to food and drink and one such reference appears in the bible. It is in the book of Daniel, where young men were being trained to be the king's servants. Daniel asked that the young men were given a ten-day try out, during which they were given only vegetables to eat and water to drink rather than the rich food of the king's court which they were expected to eat. After the ten days, the men were in better health than any of those who had remained eating the food from the royal table. This early example shows what we already understand. Fresh, simple food and plenty of water is best for our health and well-being.

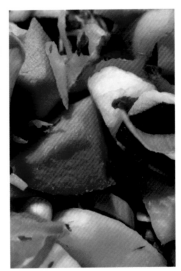

Cast your mind back to Christmas dinner. How did you feel when you were offered just another small piece of Christmas pudding or a last Belgian chocolate? How difficult was it to keep awake during your favourite television programme?

# DIET

The quote from Hippocrates at the start of this section is an interesting one. Food is not a medicine in the conventional sense, but in fact, it plays a far more important role in your natural health.

A medicine is usually brought in to deal with a problem that your body is not able to deal with itself. However, your body is actually provided with the weapons to fight off attack from all sorts of sources and the tools to repair the damage. It does this through the immune system.

When someone succumbs to an illness or disease that becomes chronic or even results in a terminal condition, then clearly the immune system is not able to do the job for which it is designed. But even lesser complaints, such as suffering from frequent headaches, colds and flu or other viruses can be a sign that the immune system is in poor condition.

So what can we do about it?

Some medicines, of course, are essential in treating illnesses. However, in those situations we should be addressing the question "Why have I become ill in the first place?" Often the answer will be found in lifestyle and above all diet.

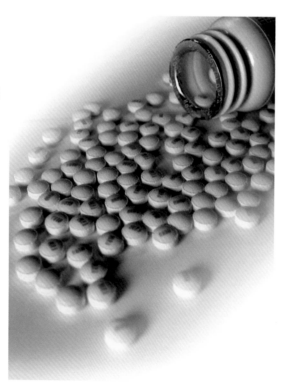

# DIET

I am not talking about going on a diet to lose weight. I am referring to everything that we eat on a daily basis.

By eating, as far as possible, those foods that provide you with all the right nutrients, you will be providing your body with all the material and energy necessary to defend itself against the stresses and toxins that we encounter and absorb throughout life. This will help you to maintain maximum health.
You will be much less likely to succumb to colds, viruses and even serious illnesses such as cancer, heart disease or diabetes if your diet contains the right amounts of vitamins, minerals and other nutrients that your body needs.

These nutrients are ideally found in fresh, unprocessed organic food.
According to the World Cancer Research Fund, "changes in diet and lifestyle could prevent 100,000 cases of cancer, each year in the UK", and that "scientists estimate that 30-40% of cancer deaths are related to diet".

Of course it is not always easy to follow such a diet on a daily basis for a variety of reasons and this is why I believe suitable nutritional supplementation as described elsewhere in this book is essential. Nevertheless, there is much we can do.

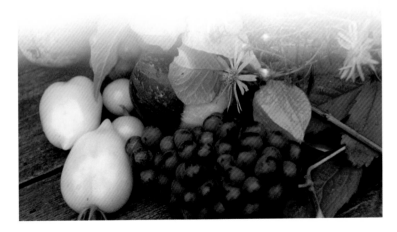

# DIET

When I talk of maximum health I do not merely mean absence of illness. What do I mean?

In his book "100% Health" which I recommend you read, Patrick Holford asks the question "are you 100% healthy with constant energy, a clear mind and freedom from pain and infection?" If you cannot say 100% yes to that question, then you need to be taking steps to make sure that you can.

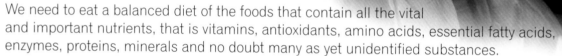

We need to eat a balanced diet of the foods that contain all the vital and important nutrients, that is vitamins, antioxidants, amino acids, essential fatty acids, enzymes, proteins, minerals and no doubt many as yet unidentified substances.

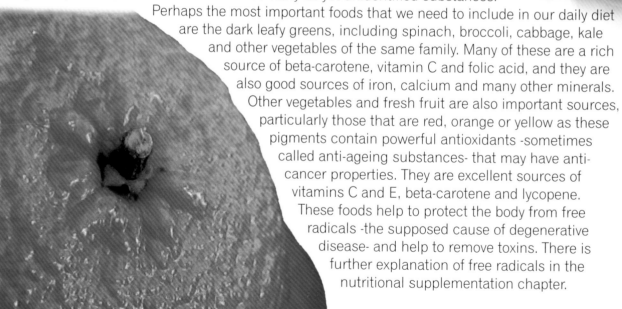

Perhaps the most important foods that we need to include in our daily diet are the dark leafy greens, including spinach, broccoli, cabbage, kale and other vegetables of the same family. Many of these are a rich source of beta-carotene, vitamin C and folic acid, and they are also good sources of iron, calcium and many other minerals. Other vegetables and fresh fruit are also important sources, particularly those that are red, orange or yellow as these pigments contain powerful antioxidants -sometimes called anti-ageing substances- that may have anti-cancer properties. They are excellent sources of vitamins C and E, beta-carotene and lycopene. These foods help to protect the body from free radicals -the supposed cause of degenerative disease- and help to remove toxins. There is further explanation of free radicals in the nutritional supplementation chapter.

# DIET

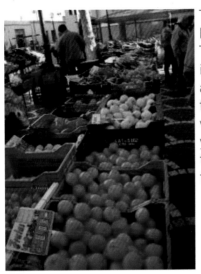

The more we eat of these foods the better, and they should be organic and as fresh as possible for maximum benefit. To be sure, much of the fruit and vegetables available to us is far from fresh and organic supplies are unpredictable and more expensive. However, we should do what we can for the good of our health. Farmers' markets may be worth visiting and if you have a garden you could grow some of your own delicious organic home produce. Re-mineralise the soil by adding volcanic rock dust to grow mineral-rich fruit and vegetables.

As I say later in the supplementation chapter, many of the fruit and vegetables can be nutritionally deficient and then, when we further reduce the vitamin and energy content by cooking, the result is food with little nutritional value. (Steaming is probably the best way to cook vegetables to retain maximum nutrition.)

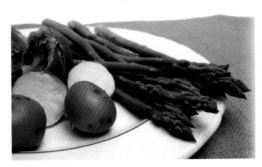

# DIET

So what is the answer?

Ideally all food should be eaten "live".
(See the Kirlian photograph of an organic vegetable exhibiting its innate energy when fresh, as opposed to cooked.)
You can eat vegetables in salads together with nuts, seeds, and beans and you will soon come to realise how delicious and satisfying they can be accompanied with dressings and fresh organic dips.

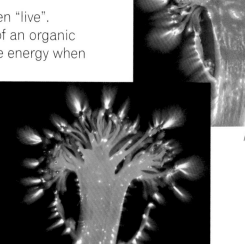

*Raw Organic Broccoli*

*Steamed Organic Broccoli*

One of my favourite juices for energy includes:

**One apple**

**One beetroot**

**Four carrots**

**One piece of celery**

**One cucumber (about 4cm)**

**Drink right away after juicing.**

There are also many interesting and simple recipes published that show different ways that you may enjoy such food. Juicing vegetables and fruit is also a great way to obtain the benefit of a greater quantity than you would easily manage, particularly when trying a range of new produce. There are some very versatile and powerful juicers now available that can produce "ice cream" from fresh frozen fruit. The blender is very useful too and, for example, soups can be made from raw vegetables that may be gently heated to allow most of the goodness to remain.

# DIET

Watch you don't overload your system with too much fruit because you can give your body too much sugar. (Fruit contains the natural sugar fructose.) Some people with poor digestion, bloating and bowel symptoms may be suffering from a yeast infection caused by an overgrowth of something called candida albicans and this fungal infection actually feeds on sugar. If you want more information on diet in relation to candida, then Erica White's "The Beat Fatigue Handbook" is worth reading. (Obviously, a qualified professional should make the diagnosis first.)

When we consume refined sugar, our pancreas produces insulin in response. When we eat a chocolate bar or have a fizzy drink, then there are what's called "sugar rushes". In our western diet we tend to add hydrogenated fats, (the fats we get in processed food), and so the pancreas can get overloaded. Is this why diabetes is on the rise?

There is conflicting evidence about the safety of aspartame in so-called diet drinks. Its better to avoid diet drinks all together. By the way, talking about chocolate, the real chocolate, made with about 70% of cocoa solids, is actually quite good for us but it must be taken in moderation.

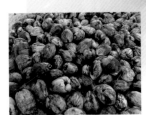

It's thought that certain substances in quality chocolate have an antioxidant effect on the body. There is also something called phenylethylamine that acts like a stimulant. We all know how chocolate can make some people feel euphoric, don't we?

Oats are something you should consider for your breakfast. As well as being nutritionally good for you they give you enough sustenance in the morning so that you should avoid snacking on junk food before lunch. I usually have organic porridge oats with flaxseeds to start my day.

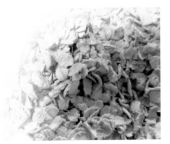

# DIET

Essential fatty acids (EFA's) are required in the diet because, as the name suggests, they are essential, but the body cannot make them. Omega 3 and Omega 6 are the EFAs to which I refer and we need to find a daily source of them in our diet.

Many people have the impression that we should eat a low-fat diet because fat is supposed to be bad for us. However the body cannot function or survive without fat.

*Did you know the brain consists largely of fat?*

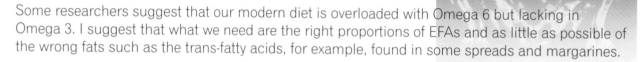

Some researchers suggest that our modern diet is overloaded with Omega 6 but lacking in Omega 3. I suggest that what we need are the right proportions of EFAs and as little as possible of the wrong fats such as the trans-fatty acids, for example, found in some spreads and margarines.

Omega 3 fats are important for their effect in reducing heart disease and building healthy brain cells. They can be found in flax seeds, walnuts and seafood, particularly in oily fish such as salmon, tuna and mackerel.

Omega 6 is needed for skin and hair growth, regulating metabolism, transporting fatty acids from the liver to the tissues and in supporting reproductive performance. Good sources can be found in corn oil, fresh nuts and seeds, sunflower seed oil and soya oil.

As I have already said, it may be important to have a proper balance of the two omegas as it seems that if the ratio is not optimised the beneficial effect is reduced.

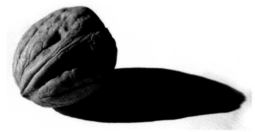

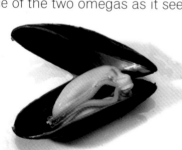

# DIET

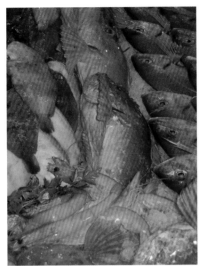

Variety in your diet is important, but for practical reasons I feel it would be a good idea to supplement with essential oils. However, we do need to be eating fresh fish two or three times a week as supplementation does not replace good wholesome food. Fish is also an excellent source of protein, vitamin B12 and iron. Similarly, nuts seeds and beans contain vitamins, protein, fibre, minerals, phytochemicals (which protect against cancer), folic acid and omega 3. Raw nuts are an ideal food source and of course they contain the natural unprocessed oil. (To revitalise nuts, just soak them for 30 minutes in water.)

Soya beans, pumpkin seeds and sesame seeds are rich in zinc and vitamin C and are a good source of protein. If using oil to cook, do not use oils that are rich in Omega 3 and Omega 6, as the effect of the heating makes them toxic. If, for example, you like to stir fry food then quickly fry in a little butter and complete the cooking using water with a water-based sauce.

"Flax and flaxseed oil are nature's richest source of omega 3's" states Professor Herb Joiner-Bay in his book "The Healing Power of Flax." Herb-Joiner Bay is an adjunct professor of classical homoeopathy and advanced therapeutics at Bastyr University, Kenmore Washington. He suggests that supplementing with essential fatty acids can reverse problems such as cracked nails, thinning hair and dry skin. " The beauty-enhancing oils (essential fatty acids) from omega-3 fatty acids and other oils (such as borage and evening primrose) are absolutely critical to the vitality and youthfulness of your skin."
(For availability of good quality essential fatty acids see information at the back of the book.)

# DIET

Whole grains are also quite nutritious but probably better not taken in excess, particularly wheat with which there is known to be a significant degree of intolerance.

On the other hand, refined carbohydrates, such as white bread, white rice and white pasta should be reduced because they are processed, incomplete foods with a reduced level of nutrition. Sometimes vitamins and minerals are added to those processed foods but, although better than nothing, these additives may not be bioavailable (able to be absorbed and utilised by the body) or in an effective proportion.

Some of the most nutritious foods are only now being recognised. These are sprouted grains and seeds. One example is bean sprouts that you may have eaten in a Chinese meal and cereal grains in the form of juice. Sprouted seeds are more easily absorbed than the seeds themselves and are much more potent. They can be grown on trays and eaten raw in salads and in the form of houmous for example.

Cereal grains, namely wheat grass and alfalfa, when harvested at the correct stage (at around eight days growth when they are at their most potent) can then be put into a specialised juicer. The resultant juice contains such a range of nutrients that it requires a book itself to fully explore all the information. There is still a lot of scientific investigation going on, but wheat grass is a wonderful regenerator and internal body cleanser and with some planning and organisation can be grown at home.

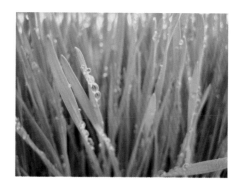

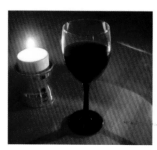

So what about wine? Are we not allowed any in our new "anti-ageing" diet? First of all, moderation in alcohol intake, and indeed in all our eating habits, is essential if we want to have energy into old age. To digress slightly, when my parents and my aunt travelled to America in the early 1990's, they used to go into a restaurant and order one steak and three plates. (Moderation again.) They have since all lived well into their 80's. But let's go back to the wine. Scientists have found that the

# DIET

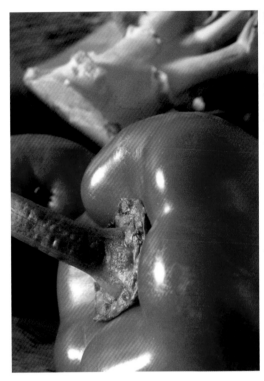

bioflavonoids present in wine may be good for you in small amounts.

One of the latest suggestions for keeping us young and healthy is for us to rebalance the pH of our blood with the foods we eat. PH is the way we measure acidity, and our blood should be slightly alkaline for maximum health. As well as breathing properly, drinking more water, reducing toxins and exercising, we can help alkalise our bodies by consuming the right foods.
(*See the information page for where to obtain alkalising green drinks*).

Examples of "alkaline foods" are more or less all vegetables, although corn is excluded since it is a grain. Most fruits are alkalising, although you should watch the quantity you take of currants, dried fruits and plums. Examples of acid foods are meat, fish, poultry, dairy products and grains. Nuts tend to be acid forming except for almonds, chestnuts, pumpkin seeds and poppy seeds. And of course alcohol and sugar ideally should be avoided if you want to experience the feeling of having a truly alkalised body. The energy you feel is staggering.

Chicken and red meats do contain many nutrients but should be eaten in smaller amounts since they can contain significant amounts of saturated fat. Meats and chicken may contain traces of chemicals resulting from the type of farming employed. Avoid any foods containing chemical additives designed to preserve, flavour or colour. As with plant foods, always attempt to obtain your meat and fish from organic or possible wild sources. That way it is easier to avoid man- made additives. That said, sources of wild fish have to be considered carefully because of environmental pollution. That is one reason, for example, for taking a patented oil blend as opposed to natural fish oil in certain circumstances.

# DIET

Your body is an amazing machine. When you embark on a diet that gives your body the correct alkalising nutrition, you actually don't crave the sugary, fatty foods that put on weight. Also, when you are mainly eating a nutritious diet, your body lets you know when you are overeating on "junk" food because it has been trained to recognise nutritious sustenance.

Another important point is that nobody has ever lived a long healthy life by eating in excess. Eating smaller meals in general is much kinder on your digestion.

When thinking about what you should be eating, bear in mind that you are approximately 75% water (see section on water) and therefore you should be trying to eat a high proportion of your diet as water based, live foods (not cooked.) This may be difficult to achieve in practice but if you keep this as your target you will be well on the way to looking better and feeling a lot healthier.

**Rules**

*Drastically reduce or eliminate processed foods including bakery, sugar and sweeteners*

*Eat in moderation*

*Avoid additives*

*Eat mainly alkaline foods*

*Eat organic foods as far as possible*

*Cooked foods should comprise only 30% of diet.*

Give yourself a treat now and again. Eat the foods that you know are not good for you in moderation but the more you alter your diet towards live, nutritious material, the more you will experience an increased energy level and a feeling of well being.

## Step 4 - Make a nutritious diet your way of life.

*Remember always to seek the advice of a qualified nutritionist if you have any queries on an appropriate diet.*

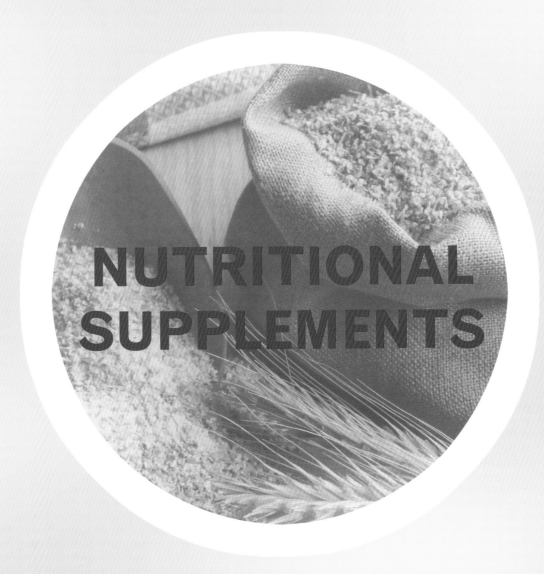

# NUTRITIONAL SUPPLEMENTS

*"The alarming fact is that food....
now being raised on acres of land
that no longer contains enough minerals
are starving us... no matter how much of
the food we eat."*

**Senate Document 264**

**The United States 7th Congress (1936)**

# NUTRITIONAL SUPPLEMENTS

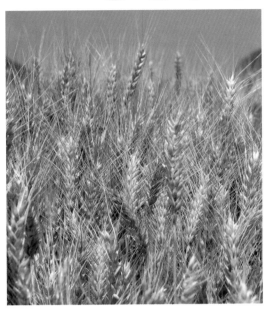

In order for your body to function properly, you probably need to provide it with at least 60 different minerals and a range of vitamins, amino acids and enzymes on a daily basis. Nature intends that we obtain these essential nutrients from our food and, ideally, a balanced and varied diet of correct food types should give us all we need.

It is recognised by many experts that, as a result of industrialised farming methods over many years, the soils, used to produce our food are producing crops that are nutritionally deficient. It may be that the soil has become demineralised or overused. This, in turn, means that many foods that we eat today contain an insufficient level of nutrients. This problem is further compounded by the use of chemicals and pesticides that, apart from the negative effects on the human body, interfere with the plants' ability to extract minerals from the soil.

We have all heard of the sailors hundreds of years ago suffering from scurvy, a deficiency of vitamin C. Vitamin C is classed as an antioxidant and there are many of these antioxidant compounds available from food. One of the most powerful antioxidants, oligomeric proanthocyanidin (OPC), present in maritime pine bark, was discovered by French scientist, Dr. Jacques Masquelier. OPCs were found to have restorative properties when used in people with nutritional deficiencies.

So why do we need plenty of antioxidants today? The human race has never had more need for them because environmental toxins are continuously attacking us. They are in the air we breathe, the water we drink, the chemicals we come into contact with and in the food we eat. Even our bodies produce toxins.

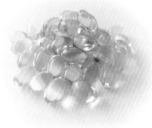

# NUTRITIONAL SUPPLEMENTS

These toxins cause free radicals to be produced and it is those that we think are responsible for ageing because they cause cellular decay and tissue damage.

Dr. Denham Harmon, a researcher from Nebraska University first proposed the free radical damage theory of ageing as the indiscriminate chemical re-activity of these molecules, possibly leading to biological changes.

If you cut an apple in two, within a few minutes you will see the cut surface turning brown. That is the effect of free radicals. Exposed, untreated steel will start to rust and this too is the same effect.

Scientists have established that human beings are capable of living healthily until 120 years or older but generally life expectancy is considered to be 70 - 80 in the Western world. Even the 70 - 80 life expectancy will often include a long period of decreased vitality and increased illness and disability.

It is thought that the cellular decay and tissue damage is responsible for at least 60 degenerative illnesses. These include heart disease, cancer, diabetes, arthritis and premature ageing.

Your body is potentially powerful and it has the mechanism to deal with free radicals, but it does need a sufficient amount of antioxidants to do the job. Not only do antioxidants allow the body to maintain its highest performance, they appear also to repair damage already caused by free radicals. This is very significant for those of us who are already suffering from the effects of such damage.

In addition to vitamin C, examples of antioxidants are vitamin E and beta- carotene. The plants we eat are beneficial for they contain bioflavonoids.

So, the question you must ask yourself is what do I want my state of wellness to be?

# NUTRITIONAL SUPPLEMENTS

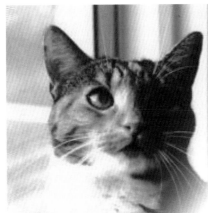

Some studies have revealed that a 40-year old has only 50% of the antioxidants in his body than would a two-year old and this deteriorates as he becomes older. Notice how much more quickly a two-year old heals or recovers from illness.

There are many reports of antioxidants benefiting a variety of conditions. Some people have even used them on their pets to good effect. This is significant because there is no evidence to suggest that the pets themselves are aware they are taking an antioxidant or being helped.

It is well accepted that many diseases are caused by the consumption of processed food. These foods have little nutritional value. (Fried foods contain a high degree of toxins caused by the heating of the oil.) Malnutrition and poisoning can follow in extreme cases. The effect is that the body does not have the ability to remove the toxins for a lack of antioxidants and minerals in the diet and the outcome is toxic overload. Disease is the result.

Apart from the toxicity of many foods we consume, another important factor is that cooking food destroys vitamins, antioxidants and enzymes. Many fruits and vegetables are far from fresh by the time we buy them and will have lost most of the nutrients that they contained. An orange, for example, that is 3 weeks old may not contain any vitamin C.

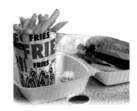

Antioxidant supplements are not medicines or drugs but are simply naturally occurring substances that should be contained in our food but for various reasons are not. Nutritional supplements are extremely effective and safe when reasonably used. Vitamins and minerals, as well as having beneficial effects individually, also work synergistically to help the body produce the appropriate substances and should always be taken together.

# NUTRITIONAL
# SUPPLEMENTS

If you are finding that wrinkles are appearing, you bruise easily, you suffer frequent colds and infections and feel groggy, then you could be experiencing the effects of a lack of the vitamins and minerals that should be provided by proper nutrition.

Vitamins such as A, C and E occur naturally in many fruits, vegetables and herbs together with bioflavonoids. These are effective antioxidants, however there are some that are much more powerful. The OPCs, as discovered by Dr Masquelier, are twenty times more effective than vitamin C in quenching free radicals. Grape seed extract is another, as well as curcuminoids (an extract of turmeric), which are three times more effective than OPCs. Curcuminoids are a must within any antioxidant supplement. That said, they all have their own unique properties and it is advisable to use a quality product containing a spectrum of vitamins, other antioxidants and herbal extracts.

An example of such a product would contain vitamins A,C,E, turmeric, ginkgo biloba, pine bark extract and grape seed extract. Taking this with the most bioavailable form of mineral supplement that can be obtained will produce the maximum effect. A good quality antioxidant should include these substances. There is a limit to what can be squeezed into one tablet and often it may be appropriate to add other individual supplements as necessary to meet your particular needs. (For details on where to obtain supplements see information page at back of book.)

Always check with a healthcare provider when taking any medication with supplements.

Many vitamins and antioxidants are water-soluble and have to be replaced on a daily basis. Vitamin C is an example of this and so it is best to take it in an esterified -- or time-lapsed-- form as this stays in the body longer.

# NUTRITIONAL SUPPLEMENTS

So what can each vitamin do?

**Vitamin E** is an antioxidant and works by protecting cell membranes against free radical damage.

**Vitamin A** is important for growth and fertility. It boosts the immune system and is essential for the normal function of vision.

**Vitamin B** comes in a variety of types. The following are some examples:

| | |
|---|---|
| **Niacin** | helps release energy from food and is important for the health of nerves and the digestive system. |
| **B6** | is essential for healthy skin, muscle and blood cells. It helps with hormone production. |
| **B12** | is necessary for the production of blood cells and the health of nerves. |

**Vitamin C** influences about 100 different enzymatic reactions and as an antioxidant, delays ageing.

**Vitamin D** is essential for promoting the absorption of calcium, which is needed for our bones.

**Oligomeric proanthocyanidins (OPCs)**, the powerful antioxidants referred to earlier, may help with diabetes, heart disease and strengthening of fragile blood vessels with improved circulation in the hands and feet.

It is important that, when taking supplements that you take the correct dose to have the desired effect. Many products are not in the most bio-available form.

# NUTRITIONAL SUPPLEMENTS

The higher the bioavailability, the more easily is it absorbed by the body. The relevance of this is that, even if the product contains a high quantity of vitamins, if they are not in a bioavailable form, the body may not absorb them easily and most of these vitamins will end up passing through the body and being flushed away. (Ask for details about effectiveness when buying nutritional products.)

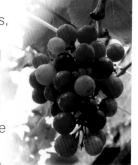

When you give your body the extra nutrition it needs by taking supplements for the first time, you may experience a mild "detox" reaction for a day or two as the body starts to release toxins. This may include a headache, colicky pain in the stomach or a skin rash. Some people say that this is a good sign -- it shows the body is starting to heal. It is particularly important at this stage to drink enough water, at least six to eight glasses a day on average to help flush out the toxins.

Even if you are not aware of any health issues, you ought to be taking antioxidants and minerals, because the body is only usually able to cope with a build up of toxins and deal with shortages of essential minerals for a certain period of time at which point a threshold is reached, often in middle age. From that point the body starts to suffer and, because a lot of damage may have been done it can take time to restore the body to its optimum condition. Furthermore, serious health issues are being identified in younger age groups as a result of poor diet and lifestyle.

In the middle ages food may have been sufficient for all our nutritional needs when soils were not overused-- but not now.

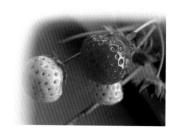

Remember we all need vitamins and minerals because these work together with the body to create good health and you can benefit by taking responsibility for yours!

**Step 5 - Consider taking nutritional supplements.**

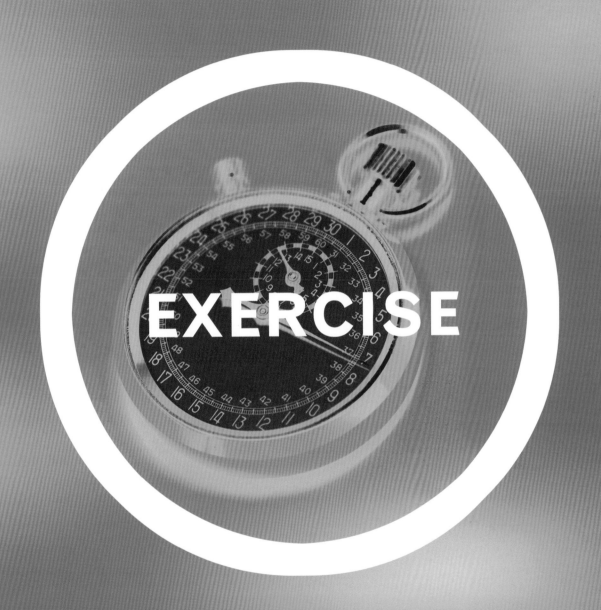

EXERCISE

*"Those who think they have not the time for bodily exercise will sooner or later have the time for illness"*

**Edward Stanley**

# EXERCISE

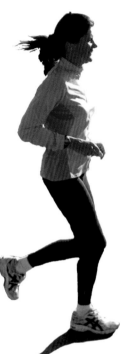

Man was meant to move but modern man does not move enough. Think about it as you get into your car, sit in front of your television or your computer.

Our modern lifestyle means that we don't have to use our muscles. We can exist indefinitely with our sedentary way of life, but we will certainly not enjoy the full potential available to us unless we utilise our bodies to the full. If you are overweight then exercise must be an integral factor in any weight-loss programme.
Exercise has got to be a way of life. It is not a programme to be taken up and set down as other more important parts of our life get in the way. We all know about walking rather than taking the car or climbing stairs instead of using the lift. Many of us are members of gyms and yet do we use our membership fully?

How can we make exercise part of our lives so that, not to take part on a daily basis would be unthinkable?

The first ingredient in anything we do is motivation.
If I was to say to you that there are two types of exercise that are guaranteed to make you look and feel younger, would that make you eager to participate? I think so. Write down all the personal reasons why you would like to feel and look better through exercise. Now write down what might happen if you never exercised. Do you want to look bloated, overweight and unable to play sport with your children or grandchildren?

The second ingredient is fun.
You must enjoy what you are doing, otherwise it just becomes a drudgery. If you enjoy dancing for example, close the blinds, put on your favourite music and enjoy the "feel good factor" as you lose your inhibitions and let your body flow. Have you ever seen the faces of some of the joggers when you know that this is really not what they want to be doing? I will tell you a way of doing 10 minutes of weight-bearing exercise indoors, which is roughly equivalent to a 30-minute jog (without the skeletal shock).

# EXERCISE

The third ingredient to successfully integrating exercise into your life is recording achievements.

Say you have never exercised before and you decide to do two minutes of exercise today. At the end of that time, write in a diary that you have successfully completed the allotted slot. For those of you who already exercise, then write down the time you have spent and mentally decide whether your goal is to increase your time tomorrow or keep to the same. Recording your success is an important part of keeping exercise integrated within your life.

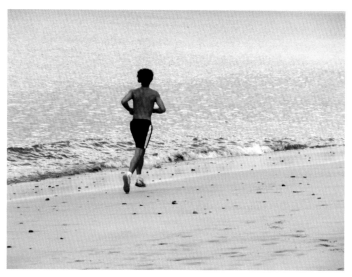

Many people will say that they don't have the time. I used to think that until I set my alarm one hour earlier in the morning in order to do some exercise before going to work. In case you are wondering, I have never been a "morning person" yet my time for exercise energises me for the rest of the day.

Always remember, before embarking on any exercise programme, get yourself checked out at your doctor's practice in case there is some medical reason you should not attempt some of the suggested movements.

There are many established practices devoted to enhancing mind/body integration. One such discipline is yoga, where the philosophy is that we should live in harmony with body and soul.

When you practice yoga under expert guidance, then you can achieve an inner stillness that enables you to listen to the signals within your body and direct energy in the body through attention and intention.

# EXERCISE

"The sun salutation" exercises are a sequence of yoga postures.
These are best performed with full consciousness as a salute to the sun. I do these exercises every morning but I have asked Julie Hanson of the Chi yoga centre to demonstrate the correct moves.

Be sure you have warmed up before doing any stretching exercises.
To warm the body, rub your hands quickly up and down the backs of your arms.
Move onto your thighs then the backs of the legs and buttocks and finally the calves rubbing vigorously.

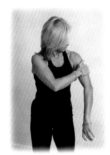 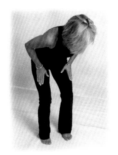 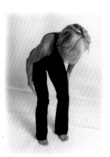

Conscious breath work is an important component of yoga and the following instructions include information on how to integrate breathing with movement:

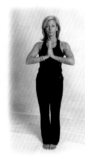

**1)** Stand upright with your feet together and inhale deeply. Exhale, then press your palms together in front of your chest, touching the skin in front of your heart with the back of your thumbs.

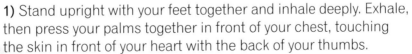

**2)** Inhale and lock your thumbs, extending your hands out in front of you. Watch your hands as you raise them high above your head and, with knees loose, not locked, lean backward from your hips as far as is comfortable.

# EXERCISE

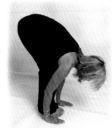

**3)** Exhale and fold your body slowly forward from the waist, bending your knees as you go down. Ideally, touch the floor with your hands but, if you are unable to do that, then let your hands hang in a relaxed manner.

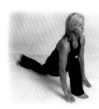

**4)** Inhale and, bending your knees, place your palms flat on the floor beside your feet. Bring your right knee up, keeping your knee at right angles to your chest and look up. Keep your right foot between your hands and extend your left foot far back and place your left knee on the floor. Bring your right knee up to your chest and look up.

**5)** Exhale and extend your right foot back to meet your left. Leave your hands where they are. Push your bottom up to make a triangle with the floor. This time look at your feet and lower your heels towards the floor.

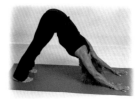

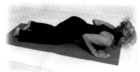

**6)** When you inhale, lower your knees, chest and chin to the floor, leaving your pelvis raised. Keep your palms beneath your shoulders and your elbows in close to your body.

**7)** Continuing to inhale, lower your pelvis to the floor and let your head and shoulder curl upward like a snake ready to attack.

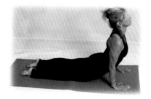

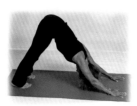

**8)** Exhale and push yourself up into the triangle position as in step five (above).

# EXERCISE

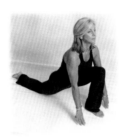

**9)** Inhale again and swing your left foot forward between your hands. Repeat as in step four but with the opposite foot.

**10)** Exhale and swing your right foot forward until it is next to the left foot between your hands. Straighten your knees while at the same time keeping your arms and hands hanging loosely or flat on the floor.

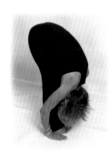

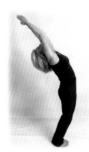

**11)** Inhale, locking your thumbs and unfolding your body slowly until you are in a standing position. Look up at your hands as you keep bending backwards as far as is comfortable.

**12)** Exhale and slowly bring your palms together in front of your chest, the thumbs touching the skin in front of your heart.

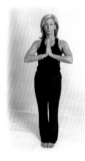

Take a deep breath and relax before repeating the exercise. Ideally, you should repeat the exercise 7 times. At the end, lie flat on your back with palms at your side facing up and listen for the controlled beat of your heart.

# EXERCISE

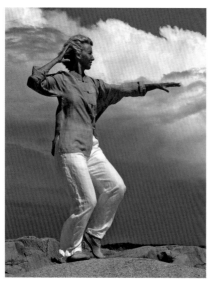

Another form of exercise, which can enhance mind/body co-ordination, is the Chinese martial art of t'ai chi. T'ai Chi involves graceful, slow movements, which improve balance, flexibility and strength, enhancing both mental and physical well-being. People who practice this form of exercise are healthier and seem younger than those who do not participate.

One of the best ways to look and feel younger is to undergo strength exercises. To build strength, you need to regularly activate your muscle groups. You need to systematically exercise the major muscle groups in your arms, legs and trunk and the key to building strength is to start off slowly and gradually build up. Holding a position for fifteen seconds provides the most benefit.

I do some exercising with a Swiss Ball. I have asked Shelley of Shelbyfit to demonstrate the use of the Ball.

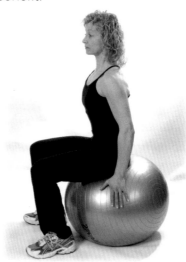

Exercising with a ball is a fun, inexpensive but a challenging way to work out. It is a great tool for addressing postural alignment and strengthening your core muscles, as well as improving balance and coordination. It is generally agreed that the better your posture, the better you function in day-to-day activities and thus lower the risk of injuries.

# EXERCISE

Warm – Up
Do not forget to warm up your muscles before starting any type of exercise as it is a way of preparing the muscles and joints for the work they are about to endure. One excellent way to warm up for both programmes of work is a fast brisk walk for about 10 minutes in order to get the large muscle groups moving as well as greater mobility for the upper body.

Lower Body
By working your lower body you will increase endurance and strengthen your leg muscles, making you less prone to injury. The more we mimic daily movements focusing on good posture the less chance we have of injuries.

Upper Body
By working your upper body you are looking to tone and strengthen your arms, shoulders and chest. Once again these exercises mimic daily activities and will help towards lifting and carrying using better posture.

Total Body
The total body exercises focus on using all the major muscle groups in your body while adding greater flexibility to your exercise programme.

## Programme One using the Swiss Ball

1. Balanced Squat Against the Wall
Place the ball against your lower back and rest it against the wall. Place your feet hip – width apart and walk your feet slightly forward pressing some body weight into the ball. Cross your arms over your chest so that your fingers rest on opposite shoulders or keep hands by your side.
Slowly bend your knees to a 90-degree angle, keeping your hips back. Your knees should stop directly over your ankles. Gently lift out of the squat and return to the start position. Repeat 10 times.

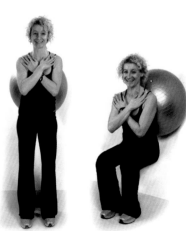

# EXERCISE

## 2. Pelvic Tilt

Sit on the ball with your back straight, with your feet flat on the floor and your hands either side. Roll backwards and forwards, keeping your upper body upright. *(This is a very small movement.)* Repeat 10 times

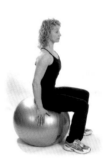

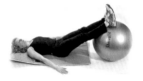

## 3. Leg Extension

Place the lower part of your legs and your feet on top of the ball. Your knees and toes should face the ceiling. Press your heels into the ball, bend your knees in towards your chest and roll the ball towards your bottom. Extend your legs out to the start position and repeat 15 times

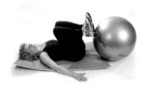

## 4. Push – Ups

Lie with the ball under your stomach and pelvis with your arms reaching the floor, shoulder width apart. Lower your chest towards the floor and push back up. Keep your body straight. Repeat 10 times.

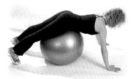

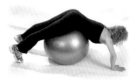

# EXERCISE

## Stretching

Stretching is a vital part of any exercise programme as it develops flexibility and lengthens the muscle fibres so any discomfort that has occurred will be eased. By becoming more flexible you are reducing the risk of injuries. As these exercises are not cardiovascular, fast or furious and fairly controlled these stretching exercises can either be used as a cool – down or interspersed within the workout.

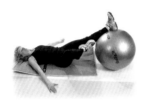

### 1. Upper Leg Stretch
Place one foot on the opposite knee. Turn the leg outwards and roll the ball towards you until you feel the stretch. Repeat 10 times on both legs.

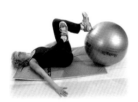

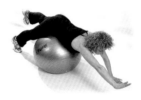

### 2. Total Body Stretch
Rest on the ball with your hands and feet on the floor. Stretch out one arm and the opposite leg and hold the position. Repeat 8 – 10 times on both sides.

# EXERCISE

## Programme Two - Exercising Without Equipment

### 1. Calf Raise

Use the stairs inside your home or a front door step and make sure your feet are parallel and are half way over the step. Use your hands for balance by either resting against the wall or banister.

Gently lift and lower your heels pushing down through your toes. Pause briefly at the top and then slowly lower. Try 10 slow repetitions.

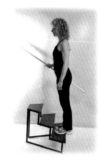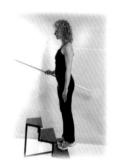

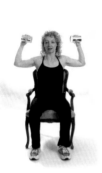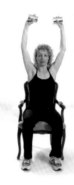

### 2. Shoulder Press

Seated on a chair imagine that the crown of your head is connected by a thread to the ceiling running up your spine. Shoulders are always down and slightly back to open up your chest. Using cans of beans, grip these in an overhand grasp with your hands a little wider than shoulder-width apart at upper chest level. Lift the weights straight up, keeping your elbows slightly bent at the top and concentrate on good posture. Lower your arms slowly back down to your chest. Repeat 10 times slowly and breathe steadily.

### 3. Chest Press

Lie on the floor with bent knees that are hip - width apart and facing forward using the cans of beans gripped in an overhand grasp as above.(Do this exercise without weights first so that you get your arms in the correct position.) Start with the weights either side of your chest with your elbows at 90°. Push the weights straight up without locking your elbows. Lower the weights slowly down to the start position.
Repeat 8 – 10 times slowly and breathe steadily.

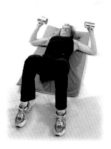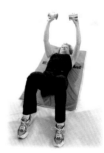

# EXERCISE

### 4. Abdominal Crunches
Lie on the floor with bent knees that are hip – width apart and facing forward. Place your arms behind your neck and contract your abdominals and curl forward, lifting your shoulder blades away from the floor. Slowly return to the start position. Repeat 10 times taking 2 to 3 seconds to lift and lower your body.

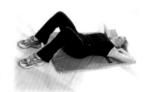

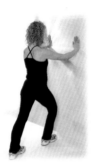

### Stretching

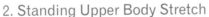

### 1. Standing Calf Stretch
Leaning against a wall in a stride stance place your arms out in front of you at shoulder height contacting the wall. Keep your head upright and looking forward, use your arms to lever ankle into a stretch and hold for 10 – 12 seconds. Repeat on both legs.

### 2. Standing Upper Body Stretch
Standing upright with legs hip – width apart place both arms overhead with hands clasped together and look straight ahead. Reach towards the ceiling to feel the stretch and hold for 10 seconds. Repeat 3 times.

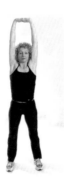

### Disclaimer
*Please ensure that you carry out these exercises in a safe environment. Shelbyfit hold no responsibility for accidents caused through misuse of the Swish Ball or carrying out an exercise incorrectly. If you are pregnant, have given birth in the last 6 weeks or have a medical condition such as high blood pressure, spinal injuries or asthma, consult your medical practitioner before beginning any exercise.*

# EXERCISE

You can store your ball inflated as long as you top up the pressure if the ball feels soft. Never over inflate your ball but make sure it feels quite firm. Clean your ball with a damp cloth and store it in a cool dry place. Avoid excessive heat.

The next type of exercise is an interesting one. It involves exercising muscles using weights for just a few seconds to produce an extraordinary increase in strength. It is called Static Contraction Training, and as strength equals youth, I suggest you check it out.

The last type of exercise I would like to mention is "rebounding." I mentioned earlier, that there is a weight-bearing exercise available indoors where ten minutes is equivalent to thirty minutes jogging. That is rebounding.

The rebounder looks like a mini trampoline but that is where the similarity ends. The best type of rebounder has a polypropylene mat--one of the strongest materials available--and a high quality steel frame and steel springs. I would recommend one with a 40-inch diameter with a height of nine inches off the floor. *(For more information on where to obtain the recommended rebounder see section at the back of the book.)*

When you first start rebounding, you must start gently if you are not used to exercise or you have a medical condition. Of course if you are fit and regularly exercise, there is a complete bodywork routine available on video that takes you through warm up and stretching exercises to intense cardiovascular conditioning.

As you rebound, you are doing what every form of exercise does for your body. You use gravity, defeating it for short periods of time as you bounce up and down. Almost everyone could be more fit by spending only a few minutes a day on a rebounder.

If you want to lose weight, then spend a few minutes rebounding before each meal since that should increase your metabolic rate. This will mean that your body will burn up your extra calories more efficiently.

# EXERCISE

The earliest report about the health aspects of rebounding came from former professional wrestler Albert Carter in a book called the " Miracle of Rebound Exercise". Trampoline artists by profession, his son and daughter took up arm wrestling and found that they were fitter, stronger and had improved balance compared with their rivals. Albert himself had a resting pulse rate of 39 that is equivalent to that of an athlete yet trampolining was the only form of exercise of which he and his family took part. He began to realise that trampolining makes use of three important forces- gravity, acceleration and deceleration. The body automatically strengthens itself to cope with the worst conditions that it repeatedly encounters.

So, with the gravity being about one and a half times the norm, rebounding harnesses this force and, as a result, the body gradually becomes stronger. NASA did some experiments on low bounce rebounders and found that they were 68% more oxygen efficient than other forms of exercise. Women in particular who should do weight bearing exercise to prevent osteoporosis should find this form of exercise beneficial.

What really interested me about 'rebounding', was the fact that people who are unable to exercise through e.g. a painful medical condition, can perform what is known as the 'therapeutic rock'. This is basically, standing with flexed knees, keeping your feet flat on the mat and gently rocking.

People who are visually impaired or have balance problems can purchase a support bar to steady them while gently rebounding. Those in a wheel chair can place their feet on the rebounder while another person bounces.

The above information is adapted from Margaret Hawkin's book about 'rebounding', which is supplied when ordering a rebounder.

**Exercise gives you energy and makes you feel better.**

**STEP 6 - Get moving.**

# EXERCISE

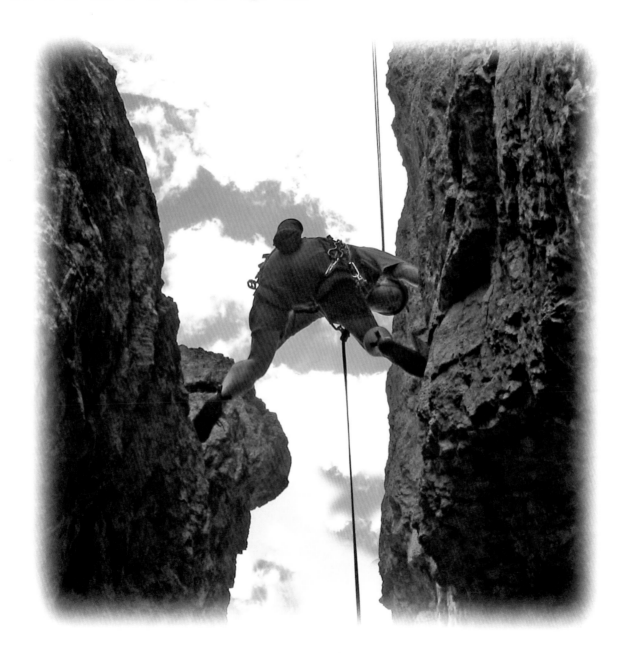

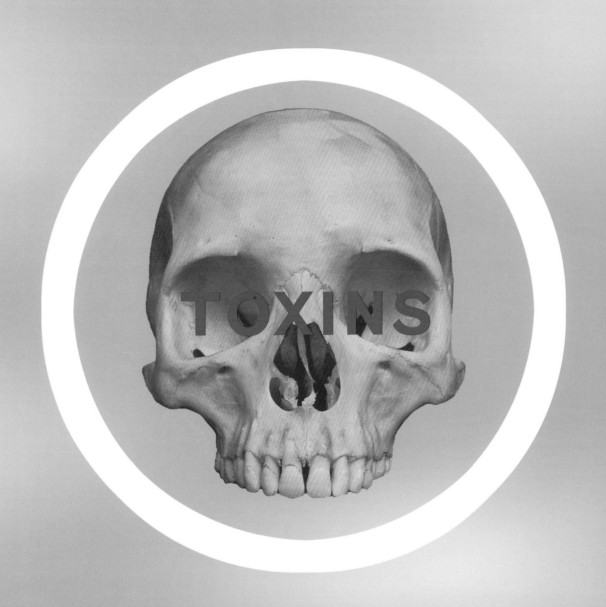

*"Slowly the poison the whole blood stream fills"*

**Sir William Epson (1935)**

# TOXINS

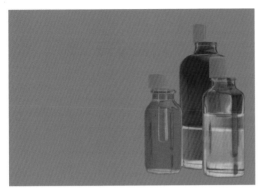

Toxins are poisons that our bodies are subjected to every day. There are environmental factors such as pollution in the air we breathe, pesticides that are used in our food industry and heavy metals in the pots and pans we use for cooking.

Some people experience a persistent headache after being exposed to the smell of fresh paint or a skin rash from a body lotion or shampoo.

Controversy surrounds the mercury fillings we have in our teeth and how that can impact on our health. It is my view that there would be an increase in mercury being absorbed by the body, should such fillings be removed. If, on the other hand, existing fillings need to be replaced then it would be worthwhile asking for an alternative material. It is important to seek expert advice on these matters from your dentist.

Clearly, excess alcohol, the toxins from cigarette smoke, caffeine and other drugs have a detrimental effect on the body. Overloading the body with foods that contain toxins, such as many of the oils that when heated become toxic *(see sections on diet and supplements)*, processed foods and additives have an adverse effect.

But what about personal care products that you use every day for washing and cleaning?

Dr. Samuel Epstein is the author of a number of publications including "The Safe Shoppers' Bible" and "Unreasonable Risk." He is chairman of the Cancer Prevention Coalition and is an internationally recognised authority on the threat of carcinogenic (cancer-producing) exposure in consumer products, including foods, household products, cosmetics and toiletries.

# TOXINS

Epstein's books list ingredients that in his opinion prove a threat to our health and it is from this information that he has recommended a company, which produces non-toxic personal care products. *(See contact information at the back of the book under toxin free products.)*

Using safe products is important since the skin is highly permeable to carcinogenic and other toxic ingredients, especially following prolonged exposure.

The potential exposure to toxic material in everyday products is great. According to daily use estimates, three personal care products are used on infants and children, men use ten products and women use six cosmetic and thirteen personal care products on average. Some are used several times a day.

Epstein believes that ingestion of toxins through the skin and mouth has a detrimental effect on our health and has the potential to increase the risk of cancer. In a supplement to its May the 8th, 2004 edition, writers at The Guardian newspaper list a catalogue of chemical compounds in every day toiletries that has the potential to affect our health.

Toxins produce an excess of free radicals in the body.

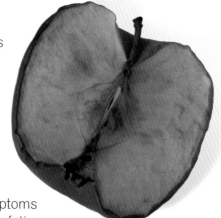

Free radicals are unpaired or unstable oxygen molecules that move in and out of cells. Your own body produces free radicals from stress, which scavenge cells and DNA (the building blocks of our bodies) looking to become stable with an oppositely charged molecule. This is an oxidative process, similar to when an apple goes brown after being cut. *(See the section on nutritional supplements.)*

Toxic overload can manifest itself in lots of different symptoms from headaches, bad breath, aches and pains to chronic fatigue.

# TOXINS

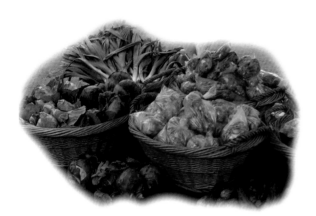

So how can we detoxify our lives?
Obviously, read the section on diet and try to increase your fresh food intake to the 70% mark.

As far as possible, always buy organic produce (without pesticides) and use fruit and vegetables when they are in season.

Imported food, stored for sometimes many weeks, will not have enough of the essential ingredients for the body to deal with toxins and the result is toxin overload and possible disease.

Increasing our water and oxygen intake is another important way to detoxify.
(*See Steps 2 and 3*).

Many health food shops sell detoxification kits but I would recommend that the detoxification is performed in a controlled manner with the correct liquid nutrients taken as part of the cleanse.
(*For more information, see our website* www.newlifehealthcare.co.uk )

Our bowels harbour toxic waste materials that the body must eliminate to remain healthy.

Processed foods and those with little fibre reduce transit time in our bowels and, as such, build up toxins that can inevitably lead to disease.

The bowel was not designed to deal with chemical additives, artificial colouring and flavouring, but it copes most efficiently on fresh fruits, vegetables, grains, nuts and seeds.

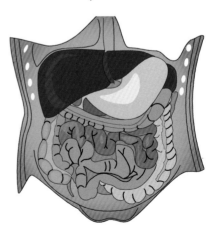

# TOXINS

Dr John Tilden, in his book "Toxaemia Explained", suggests that disease emanates from toxins contained in the bowel.

Colonic irrigation-- which means flushing out the bowel with warm water-- remains controversial, but to detoxify completely there needs to be an adequate clear out of all toxic material.

It is thought that the bowel contains 10-15lb of faecal material at any one time and that regular elimination-- after each meal-- is necessary to reduce toxic overload.

If you do want to try colonic irrigation then always check the status of the practitioner. Remember, your doctor might not agree.

The lymphatic system plays a major part in cleansing the body tissues and drainage of the waste products. This system is a type of secondary circulation that is intertwined with the blood supply.

Lymph is the basic material, which is plasma, after it has exuded from the capillaries. Bathing the cells, it brings nourishment and takes away the waste material. The lymphatic system doesn't have its own pump but must work efficiently for health so stimulating the system will improve immunity and increase energy levels. Examples of problems that cause a restriction in lymphatic flow are chronic dehydration, prolonged rest periods, nerve lesions and inflammation.

Increasing lymphatic flow helps to detoxify the body.
One of the simplest ways to do so is to partake in regular exercise.
*(See section on exercise.)*

Brisk walking and swimming are two examples where contracting skeletal muscles stimulate the flow of lymph.

# TOXINS

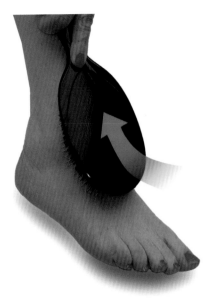

Dry skin brushing removes the dead surface skin and is an effective method of increasing lymphatic flow.

The brush used needs to be of natural bristle and kept dry.

Before showering or bathing, start brushing the skin from the feet.

Each stroke should be like a clean sweep always in the direction of the heart.

After the feet, brush up the legs and the buttocks then the hands, arms and down the neck and trunk.

For the shoulders and upper back, brush across the top so that exactly the right pressure is applied.

Use skin brushing every day if possible but a minimum of three times a week to not only exfoliate the skin leaving it softer but also as a form of detoxification.

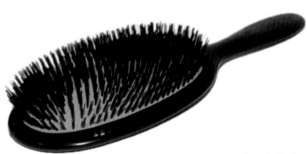

For details of availability of
Detox Bristle Brush
*(See further information at the back of the book.)*

# TOXINS

Deep breathing *(as in the section on oxygen)* oxygenates the tissues while the movement of the diaphragm helps stimulate lymphatic flow.

Rebounding *(see section on exercise)* is an excellent way to boost the lymphatic system. A simple movement where you stand on the mat, feet flat and gently rock
is particularly useful for those with painful and debilitating conditions.

A specialised massage technique called lymphatic drainage treatment is useful for detoxifying the body. It requires the special skill of a trained therapist with or without the use of aromatherapy oils to re-energise you.

Everything in this section will help you to eliminate -- or certainly reduce-- the level of toxins in your body. Pick two or three methods and make a start to make yourself look better and dramatically increase your energy levels.

**STEP** 7
**- Reduce the toxins
  in your body.**

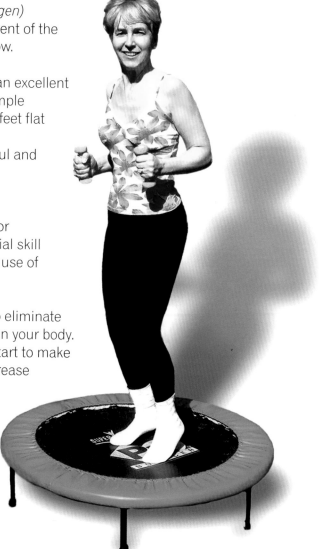

# RELATIONSHIPS

*"The true measure of a man is how he treats someone who can do him absolutely no good"*

**Samuel Johnston**

# RELATIONSHIPS

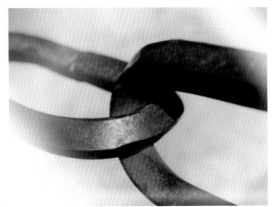

Relationships are probably the most important part of your life. When other things go wrong, as they inevitably will, the anchor of solid, dependable and lets not forget exciting relationships form the steadying as well as the energising influence in what we want out of life.

Have you ever wondered why you don't get on with certain people yet there is no apparent reason why this is so? I want you to think of someone now that frankly irritates you. Then I want you to think about three traits that you can identify as the main reasons for that irritation. Think seriously about these traits and once you have done so you will realise that you may actually have similar characteristics. Amazing, isn't it?

The good thing is that you now have the chance to change. Watch as other people warm to you and notice that you will get along with a far greater number of people.

It took me a long time to realise that the way you speak to someone has a lot to do with whether you can effectively communicate.

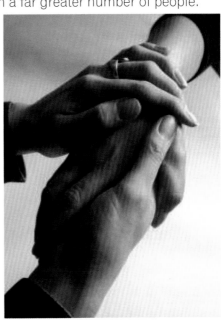

We can loosely categorise people into archetypes. These categories describe our most dominant trait and personality type.

We would include our natural inclinations, strengths and weaknesses, and this determines how we naturally respond in most situations.

# RELATIONSHIPS

Some examples are the "tiger" personality type who is a born leader. He is confident, self-reliant and tends to take charge of any situation.

Problems can arise because the naturally dominating trait means that the type of communication used is normally forceful, sometimes blunt and impatient. If this "tiger" personality is talking with a "lamb" type personality--someone who is timid, diffident and sensitive-- then the communication will fail.

The first thing you should do to maximise the effectiveness of communication when talking with someone is to model both their body language and the tonality of their voice. If a person speaks very softly and slowly and you talk to them in loud impatient tones then they basically will not like you.

If on the other hand you become aware of the way they are speaking and try to emulate them in a very caring way, suddenly you will find they will want to continue the communication. I'm sure you can think of examples where that scenario would be very useful.

People do not tend to notice if you sit the same way as they do and use similar hand gestures and facial expressions. What happens is that a complete stranger will warm to you if you take note of their body language and act similarly.

Of course body language generally can impact greatly in any communication. The obvious signals of body language--looking at your watch or having your arms folded while talking with someone-- will not create the correct impression.

On the other hand, an open pose with a similar stance as the person with whom you are talking will greatly improve mutual empathy.

# RELATIONSHIPS

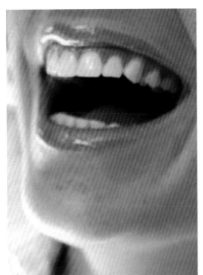

Next time, when a shop assistant gives you your change or a waitress brings you the food you ordered, engage them in some conversation. Most people wear name badges so, since most people like to hear their name being spoken, say their name and ask them a question maybe about when they started work that morning. Depending on the answer, you can perhaps sympathise with them and watch the difference in how you are treated next time you ask for something.

There was a group of English tourists travelling across Europe with a tour operator. One couple decided to check before they travelled as to how to communicate with all the different nationalities of the people they would encounter since they had no knowledge of foreign languages.
A seasoned traveller gave them one piece of advice--treat everyone you meet with a high degree of respect. As the tour progressed, the couple noticed that they were given the best rooms in each hotel and never had any problem at meal times whereas others in the party, who were loud and impatient with staff, seemed to attract a catalogue of disasters with accommodation and service along the route.

To have good relationships, you must master listening skills.

No one really listens to another person. It is an art and it can also be learned. How do you feel when someone you are talking with is looking over your shoulder, eyes darting, interrupting what you are saying? I suggest, either annoyed or hurt.

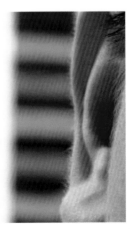

On the other hand, watch a parent who is listening lovingly and intently to her child. How does that child feel when that happens?

# RELATIONSHIPS

A young man was lucky enough to sit beside two eminent American politicians at two separate dinners in Washington. The first dinner involved Richard Nixon and afterwards he was asked what it had been like. He answered that he thought Nixon was the most interesting person in the world.

At the second dinner, he sat beside John F Kennedy. Once again he recounted his impressions of the evening and this time he said that Kennedy made him feel that he, the young man, was the most interesting person in the world.

The key to good relationships is to be interested rather than interesting. It's difficult when you meet someone with whom you have little in common to find something of interest in what they are saying. Start to imagine they are the most interesting person you have ever come across, listen, ask questions and soon you will be wrapped up in their conversation.

Once, there was a businessman working for a large industrial chemical plant who travelled all over the world meeting chief executives and government officials in many countries. The businessman was a "loner" and, in the hotel lounges he used to sit as far away from other guests as possible when he stayed the night.

One night, after dinner, he positioned himself at the far corner of the bar but unfortunately, or so he thought, a stranger approached him and introduced himself. This stranger just loved to talk to people and started to ask the businessman a lot of questions. The businessman responded warily at first but realised that this person was just a traveller like himself whom he would probably never see again.

After about an hour the stranger excused himself as he was beginning to feel quite jaded. The businessman stopped the stranger and said to him, "You know, you are the most interesting person I have ever met." The stranger thanked the businessman and said goodnight. After walking away the stranger thought to himself, "I only told the businessman my name!"
Treat the other person you are with as the most important person on earth and watch your relationships soar.

*The above example is adapted from Jay Abraham's 'Your Secret Wealth.'*

# RELATIONSHIPS

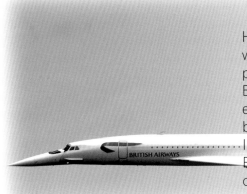

Have you ever surprised someone? The enjoyment comes when you see the surprise on the face of the individual-- what pleasure that is both for yourself and the person involved. Betty used to work with my father for many years and eventually ended her working career with me in my own business. When it came to her retirement, I knew I wanted to do something special to mark the occasion. For several months before the date I listened carefully to the conversation Betty had about what she might do when she was retired. One of the things that kept cropping up was a trip on Concorde, and so I started plotting a surprise for her.

I found out there was a trip to the Baltic leaving from Heathrow, and to mark the occasion I thought it would add a touch of class if Betty was picked up from her house and driven to the airport in a chauffeur-driven Rolls Royce.

My father's 80th birthday party seemed a good time to present her with the two tickets and I'll never forget the look on her face as she realised what was involved. (She was to choose her partner for the day and decided it was to be her husband.)

The day approached and the photographer from the local newspaper arrived to capture the moment when they headed off in their limousine.

Betty recounts phoning her friend from Heathrow with the words "must dash, I'm about to board Concorde."

It was champagne all 'round on board, and when Betty finally came down to earth she was able to recount just how that experience was so amazing for her.

Of course, now that Concorde is no longer flying commercially, her memory is even more special.

# RELATIONSHIPS

Another example of the excitement and pleasure of surprise was when my parents held their golden wedding. I decided to hold a "This is Your Life" party with a friend from my drama club, Walter, playing the part of presenter Michael Aspel, and of course all the planning had to be done in secret!

Months before the event I talked with all the people who had been involved with my parents at --and since-- their wedding day.

I recorded their stories on audio-tape. One of my mother's bridesmaids recalled the time when everyone in the bridal party retired to the vestry to sign the register, then ended up going through the floor followed by hoots of laughter. The wedding had been held in an old church in Ireland and the vestry floor had not been maintained to receive the weight of nine adults.

The guests for "This is Your Life" were given strict instructions not to park their cars near our house, and even the firm that was to deliver the extra chairs for the event were sent next door the day before in case my mother arrived unexpectedly at our house.

I had arranged a surprise lunch at a restaurant for the day of the golden wedding. My parents thought the excitement of the day was over as we headed back to our house. It was very late by this time as my mother had first wanted to go and see her old school and beach where she had played as a young girl.

Meanwhile, back at the house people were shut away in the various rooms waiting to be called in at the appropriate time.

My parents were flabbergasted and delighted when "Michael Aspel" met them as they approached the door of the house and presented them with the famous red book and the immortal words "Betty and Jimmy--this is your life." Meeting all their old friends and relations was such a pleasure to watch. Have you got an idea of a surprise for someone close to you?

# RELATIONSHIPS

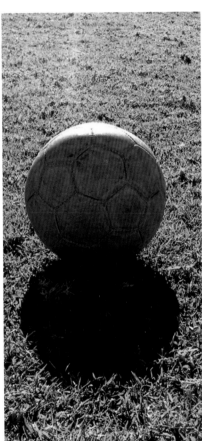

How can we influence our partners or children in a constructive, beneficial way and create the sort of relationships we want? The following is a story of the power of beneficial influence adapted from Stephen Scott's "Mentored by a Millionaire".

The big love of Dan's life was football. He loved to play with an amateur team at weekends and would have been a professional but for an injury he had sustained as a teenager. During the week he was a successful computer analyst and travelled extensively for his world-renowned company.

His lady friend was called Carry and he had got engaged to her at the age of 40, but still, two years later, had not set a date for the wedding. Carry loved Dan very much and had such a delightful nature that Dan's friends joked with him that if he didn't hurry up and marry her then one of them would.

Dan and Carry were both Christians and their relationship was so pure that they didn't want to live together before marriage and were willing to wait. This was very difficult for Carry since she loved Dan so much and wanted to be his wife and be the mother of his children. She also knew that marriage was right for Dan as well.

The problem was that the waiting went on and on. Dan was a loving man and fun to be with, but he couldn't commit to marriage. Carry realised that she would have to help Dan feel how she was feeling in the relationship for him to commit, so she thought deeply about his life.

# RELATIONSHIPS

When Dan went along to play football he was quite often relegated to the bench. Carry knew that he felt downhearted and frustrated at the manager's decision because he practised hard, and when he was asked to play, he often scored a goal.

Carry decided to talk to Dan one Saturday night at dinner after he had failed to be asked to play once again by the manager. She asked Dan: "How do you feel when you realise you're once again relegated to the subs bench on a Saturday afternoon?" He then started to recount all his usual frustration, disappointment and unhappiness. She then turned this around to their relationship and explained to Dan that that was how she felt. It was like being relegated to the subs bench waiting to get married!

Dan just couldn't believe what he was hearing. He could now feel what she was feeling. He felt exactly the same way on a Saturday afternoon when his manager read out the first-team names and his was not among them. Dan set the date for the wedding that night and everything moved quickly from then on.

Dan wondered why he had waited so long as it was a lot of fun to plan the wedding. Who was going to sit beside Auntie Jess and should they invite cousin Bert who they hadn't seen in years? What type of house were they going to live in? It wasn't as if Dan had to be forced into marriage. He had suddenly realised what he was missing.

Can you see the powerful use of influence to benefit both people in a partnership?

Can you think of an example in your own life to make a relationship better?

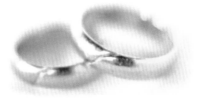

# RELATIONSHIPS

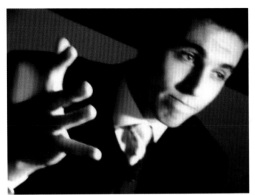

You must honour the other person's point of view, listen and understand first, then pick both the right moment and the right topic to make the other person feel what you are feeling.

I'm sure many women can identify with the scenario where the female partner comes back from work. Mary's had a bad day and simply wants to unburden the story onto her partner. Bill, on the other hand, is sitting reading the paper and can't understand what all the fuss is about.

The conversation may go something like this:

**Mary:** That's it. I've had enough of Barbara at the office. She just doesn't understand what my priorities are. I might as well not bother.

**Bill:** Well why don't you just quit?

**Mary:** What do you mean quit? I've worked for years in that office to get the things the way they should be--what a stupid suggestion.

**Bill:** What do you mean stupid? It seems to me that you're constantly moaning about your work and you'd be much happier in another office.

You can see the way this conversation is going and, really, it's a male/female "lack of understanding of the differences in communication" that is the cause of the argument.

131

# RELATIONSHIPS

Men need to understand that that they have to listen and let her rant and rave with suitable noises such as "oh no" and "yes, I understand" to make the relationship work.

Women, on the other hand, must realise that men want to fix things. They want to offer a solution to her problem, so to call his suggestion to quit stupid is like showing a red matador's cape to a bull.

Men need to be respected while women need to be emotionally understood. Dr John Gray explains these differences in an extremely entertaining way in his book "Men are from Mars Women are from Venus".

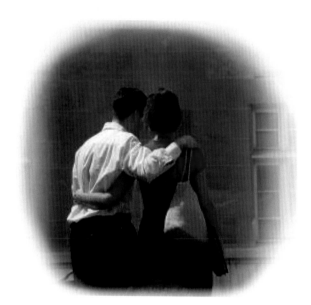

Spend some time to learn about the different communication skills between men and women and your relationship will significantly improve.

But what about someone reading this that isn't in a relationship but would like to be? Is it possible to think yourself into a relationship?
The first thing you have to do is close your eyes and imagine the person you would like as your mate. The more detail you can bring to your mental picture the better.

The next thing you have to do is make a list of all the attributes that your ideal mate requires. It's important to add enthusiasm to each trait. The more excitement you add and "feel" that feeling inside, the greater will be the move towards your desired outcome.

# RELATIONSHIPS

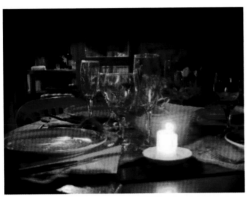

Now let us examine the practical side. Look around at the night classes available in your area or choose a sport that has mixed players. Tell your friends that you are on a quest to find your ideal mate— it's amazing how they will come up with ideas or even invite you to dinner with "suitable" people that usually are totally unsuitable! Don't despair, since at least your social life is now picking up and if you visualise and think about your partner every day then he/she will turn up when you least expect it.

But there is one vital ingredient you need to include in this process. You have to become the person that will attract your ideal mate. If you are a woman who is severely overweight, then you can't expect to attract someone that looks like George Clooney. You can, of course, do something about your weight if you organize a plan of only eating nutritious food and exercising every day. How about it?

Now what about relationships that seem to be withering on the vine? We can all look back to that time when we met someone and there seemed to be a spark, a sexual chemistry that excited us whenever we thought about that person.
He or she could do no wrong in our eyes, and when family or friends pointed out any imperfections we were hugely defensive. When you live with someone for a long time -- either in marriage or as partners-- many people forget or don't even know about the important communication skills that are needed to keep a relationship fully alive. Criticism of each other's habits tends to be the only communication made, apart perhaps from talk about the children.

Look around a restaurant next time you are out and see if you can spot the "tired" relationships where the couple are sitting in silence compared with the animated chatter of a relationship that is working well.

# RELATIONSHIPS

If you identify with the former couple, what can you do to recharge that excitement in the relationship?

First of all, can you appreciate there are different types of language that separates us from each other?

Take for example the wife who receives chocolates and flowers from her husband but secretly thinks they are a waste of money. What she really wants is her husband's praise and support for her ideas-- ideas that she is gathering for a new venture she is starting now that the children have left home. He, on the other hand, thinks the flowers and chocolates are an important physical symbol of his love for her and he has no conception that what she really wants is his support.
Another example might be that the husband is a workaholic and his wife doesn't seem to be able to spend any time with her spouse. Although he provides all her monetary needs, he is excluding her from his time. Gradually, they drift apart until they are barely communicating.
It may seem obvious but one of the things you can do is write down all of the attributes of your other half and start to tell each other those that you admire.

In the first example the wife might state that verbal support from her spouse is the most important trait, whereas the husband might say that to be appreciated ---not because he brings her chocolates, but because he is always there for her-- might start to bring the relationship alive.

In the second example quality time spent with each other is often forgotten in the rush of everyday responsibilities and seeing to the children. Spend 15 minutes a day just listening to each other-- no television or reading newspapers-- just giving each other undivided attention.
Take the case of the workaholic. What does his wife like to do, and could he accompany her on these activities? Just doing these two things with his wife while she, on the other hand, praises him for doing well at his job and providing for the family could make an enormous difference to their lives.

# RELATIONSHIPS

In another relationship, there may be problems where one of the partners never helps around the house. I'm afraid it is usually the male so I will use that in the next example.

Simon's mother did everything for him before he was married. He naturally assumed that his wife Sarah would do the same when they got married. That was the start of their problems, because Sarah had always been an independent woman and had a cleaning lady to help in her flat when she was single.

As their marriage began to flounder, they attended a marriage counsellor who asked each of them separately to make a list of what tasks need done around the house and who should do each. Four of the tasks on each list were assigned to each person and both realized that, to make each other happy it would only require a small shift in the working relationship. That list probably saved their marriage.

Physical touch can be an important "language" in any relationship. If one of the partners fails to recognize this, then the relationship can run into trouble.

When the female is crying it may be critical that her partner comforts her with physical touch. He needs to know his partner's needs.

The female in the relationship needs an emotional base before she can truly appreciate the physical side of the marriage, whereas it is generally the male domain to show his feelings for his partner through the physical act of sexual intercourse.

If the female feels loved and appreciated by her partner then she will want to be intimate. The emotional side of her "being" often determines her physical desire. In a relationship where the physical side is no longer of such importance, then both parties have to examine their emotional and physical needs separately and then together.

# RELATIONSHIPS

The last subject in the chapter on relationships is that of sales. I don't just mean physical products but it may mean that you have to "sell" your idea to a club committee, a family member or a spouse.

In my first example, let's say you have an ideal holiday plan that involves a lot of your favourite sport but your partner wants to spend some time with his or her elderly mother while your children are looking for a beach holiday.

That sounds like an impossible task to please everybody. Of course you could just go ahead and book your holiday. I suggest that wouldn't add a lot to the relationship, or you can spend some time looking at how to arrange a compromise.

Get some brochures and a large sheet of paper. Hold a family conference and write down everything that everyone wants to do. Look at the places available and plan to visit an area that can accommodate everybody's wishes. This example is looking at negotiation skills, but in terms of relationships I'm sure you can see how family relationships can only improve.

Try this idea with any plan that involves people reaching a difficult decision and see how well it works.

What about when you have to sell either a product or maybe a concept to a business firm? The first thing you have to do is develop a relationship with the people in the firm. We have all been subjected to a salesperson that has been completely out of tune with our thinking and, even if we wanted the product, we would never buy because of that particular individual. It may take several months to build up rapport with a firm.

Who are the decision makers? Is their a receptionist or secretary that can influence decisions even concerning access to key individuals?
One such salesman called on a firm several times never making a sale but always just reminding the people he interacted with at each visit what benefits he could offer them. His patience paid off and after some time, he was awarded a very lucrative contract, which would never have come about if he hadn't painstakingly nurtured the relationship.

**STEP 8 - Get your relationships in order and feel a lot better.**

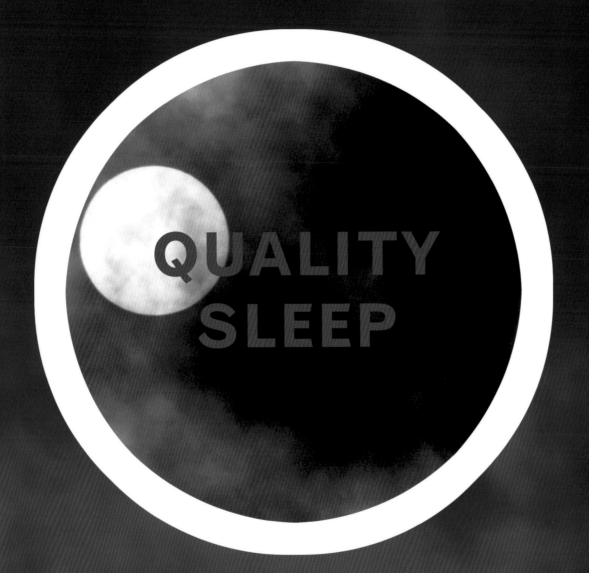

QUALITY
SLEEP

"Now, blessings light on him
that first invented sleep!"

**Don Quixote**

# QUALITY SLEEP

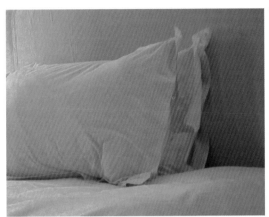

The best way to revive your mind and body is through quality sleep. What do we mean by quality sleep? My definition is when you feel rested and able to get on with your tasks within a few minutes of rising. If you practice meditation, the time to do it is just after awakening-- preferably at dawn.

There are different stages of sleep starting with our brains "switching off" wakefulness and activating our sleep centres. I'm sure, like myself, you have experienced the "falling off a cliff" type of sensation when starting to sleep, that is quite normal but it usually goes unnoticed in sleep.

The stimulated beta waves of our brain's electrical activity during the day should now have changed to the much slower alpha waves --called relaxed wakefulness-- and as we become drowsier the alpha waves become interspersed with the even slower theta and delta waves.

The "rapid eye movement" (REM) stage of sleep shows our brains as highly active, yet our muscles-- except those that are essential to life-- are paralysed. REM sleep is where we dream and it is thought that dreaming is particularly important in our overall emotional well-being.

About 50% of our sleep is spent in light sleep. In deep sleep the body can repair blood cells, body tissues and even the brain.

# QUALITY SLEEP

To feel well and energised requires us to have a complete, uninterrupted sleep, covering all stages of sleep.

It is believed that dreaming can be used to solve problems.
Do our dreams mean anything? First of all do you remember your dreams?
Unless you are disturbed during the night during a particularly vivid dream, then you probably will have no recollection of even having had a dream.

If you want to use the information contained in your dreams, you first have to write down any dream on paper when you do recall one. Usually the dream description will make no sense, however the more dreams you write down the better you will be able to link the concepts to something in your life.

There are some people who have trained their minds to such an extent that they can programme themselves to recall their dreams and others who give their mind a problem to solve before falling asleep. The command on this occasion is to remember and understand the dream so that the solution will be ready for you in the morning. During this dreaming time, in our sleep pattern, the conscious part of our brain is negated and therefore we are somehow contacting the unconscious or higher, inspirational aspects of our mind.

I'm sure we have all experienced the problem that seemed insurmountable the night before, paling into insignificance in the morning after we have obviously worked it out during our sleep cycle.
If you have a faith you can use the time just before sleep to pray for help with a difficult problem.

In experiments, people who kept being woken up every time they entered the REM sleep phase became irritable, vague and easily tired. Quality sleep is a must for good health, and to reach our maximum potential try writing down your dreams then interpret them and see what happens.

# QUALITY SLEEP

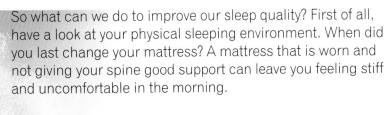

So what can we do to improve our sleep quality? First of all, have a look at your physical sleeping environment. When did you last change your mattress? A mattress that is worn and not giving your spine good support can leave you feeling stiff and uncomfortable in the morning.

What about the temperature of the room? A good bedroom temperature should be 62°F.(16.6°C) Noise when falling asleep can have both an annoying and a soothing effect. The sound of waves crashing against rocks can relax you but the dripping sound of a tap can leave you unable to sleep.

Feng Shui is the ancient Chinese art of balancing two forces known as yin and yang so that the life force--qi--can be harmonised in our environment. That environment in the bedroom should be both relaxing for sleep and energising for waking. Get yourself a book on Feng Shui in order to physically balance your bedroom surroundings.

Don't eat close to bedtime since that will put your digestive system into overdrive. Leave at least three hours before retiring after consuming a large meal. It's suggested that tyramine, a protein in cheese, stimulates chemicals in the blood stream that can cause high blood pressure and therefore the feeling of stress when we experience a nightmare.

Magnesium in foods such as green vegetables, avocados, nuts, seeds and bananas has been shown to improve the quality of sleep. It's the same--but true--story about a balanced, nutritious diet and eating smaller meals throughout the day that aids restful sleep.

Remember to drink extra water before bed if you have taken any alcohol because dehydration can affect sleep. Alcohol in small amounts can have a relaxing effect but larger amounts can produce a restless night by reducing the amount of REM and deep sleep.

# QUALITY SLEEP

Winding down before bed is important. Everyone enjoys a good thriller, but try to avoid violent or graphic television late at night because the visual stimulation excites the nervous system. That, of course, is the direct opposite of what you require at night. Obvious stimulants such as caffeine-- remember they are contained in some soft drinks as well as coffee and tea—can adversely influence sleep. On the other hand, a few drops of lavender oil on your forehead or pillow will induce a restful state.

What about exercise in relation to sleep? Have you ever experienced going for a long walk either in the country or by the sea and finding yourself, about 9 o'clock that night, nodding, ready to sink into a wonderfully deep sleep? Our modern lives generally don't include that sort of healthy exercise, so if you have a sedentary lifestyle then it might be worthwhile stretching your spine in an exercise before bed. (Obviously, if you have an injury or are pregnant, seek professional advice before trying the following exercise.)

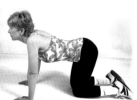

Attempting a cat like stretch involves going onto all fours with your hands flat on the floor directly under your shoulders and your knees directly under your hips. Inhale, lift your head up and push your bottom out at the same time as dipping your back. Exhale and breathe steadily while holding that position for 30 seconds. The second stretch involves the same initial position on all fours and, while breathing in, lower your head to look between your legs. As you breathe out, tuck your chin into your chest, arch your back upwards and tuck in your bottom. Maintain this position for 30 seconds while breathing steadily. Hopefully, the stress and tension built up over the day will be released, enabling you to fall asleep more easily.

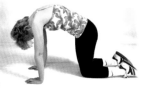

Massaging the soles of your feet with something like sesame oil can promote sound sleep. The feet are said to contain many points that relate to a balancing of the nervous system. Warm the oil before use and after a minute or so it can be washed off with a damp cool cloth. This will create a soothing effect in preparation for sleep.

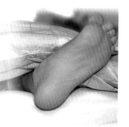

# QUALITY SLEEP

Sometimes we have prepared ourselves well for sleep yet it eludes us.
Is there anything that can be done to help? First re-read the problem-solving paragraph on dreams and try that method if you are worrying about something.

Another way of helping you get to sleep uses the Silva Method. The method uses a simple, step-by-step approach to teach you to function at an inner conscious level helping you to become more creative and with enhanced intuition.

I attended a Silva Method workshop where the instructor explained the "chalk board" exercise for promoting sleep. With your eyes closed, breathe out fully three times while mentally repeating and visualising the numbers 3, 2 and 1 in sequence. Practice relaxing each part of your body. Start with your head and work down. If you haven't fallen asleep by this time, visualise a chalkboard.

"You will have chalk in one hand and an eraser in the other. You will then mentally draw a big X within the circle. You will then proceed to erase the X from within the circle, starting at the centre and erasing towards the inner edges of the circle, being careful not to erase the circle in the least. Once you erase the X from within the circle, to the right and outside of the circle you will write the word "deeper", and you will tell yourself that you are entering a deeper, healthier level of mind, in the direction of normal, natural, healthy sleep.

You will then write a big number 100 within the circle; then you will proceed to erase the number 100 being careful not to erase the circle in the least. Once the number 100 is erased, to the right and outside of the circle you will go over the word "deeper". Every time you go over the word "deeper", you will tell yourself that you are entering a deeper, healthier, level of mind, going in the direction of normal, natural, healthy sleep.

You will continue using the numbers within the circle on a descending scale until you enter normal, natural, healthy, physiological sleep."

# QUALITY SLEEP

As you probably realise this is an extremely boring task, and what happens to us when our brains do not have enough to do? Yes, we feel tired so, hopefully, this method will get you off to sleep without too much trouble. *(For contact details on the Silva Method, see information page.)*

Let's finish with the steps for promoting quality sleep:

- Review your physical surroundings as well as your bed.

- De-stress yourself with stretching exercises or massage.

- Give your mind your most challenging problem by asking yourself to solve it in your dreams or try the "chalkboard" method.

- Eat sensibly in the evening, avoiding stimulants such as coffee.

- Stop watching television at least an hour before bed.

If you experience quality sleep on an ongoing basis, you will feel better during the day and will experience more energy.

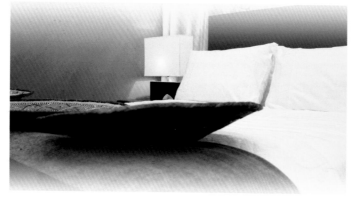

**STEP 8  Get some quality sleep.**

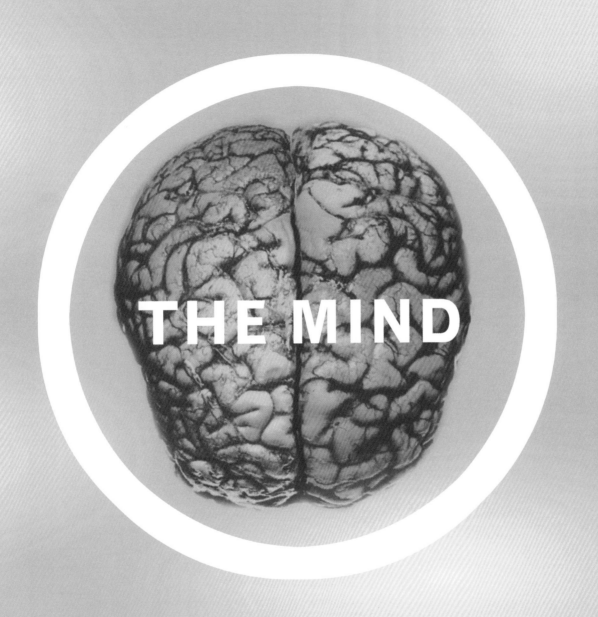

# THE MIND

"There are more things in heaven and earth Horatio
than are dreamt of in your philosophy"

**William Shakespeare (Hamlet)**

# THE MIND

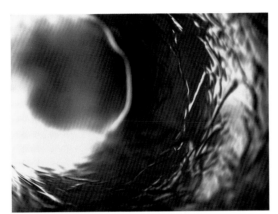

The mind is a field of energy that we experience subjectively. Unlike the body, which is made up of molecules, the mind is made up of ideas.

Every living being emits light in the form of photons. As mentioned in the diet section of the book, if you look at a Kirlian photograph of a human or a plant (particularly an organic plant), there is an aura of light around each form. The photographs capture the electromagnet radiation patterns emitted by objects across a wide spectrum of electromagnetic energy.

In a sense what we reflect out to the world is reflected back to us.

How many people remember being 16 and in love? We had a permanent smile on our faces, nothing was too much trouble and life couldn't have been better. When you experience happiness you have more energy and direction in your life. We'll rate that state of happiness around the 90% on a scale of 0 - 100.

At the other end of the scale, I want to tell you about Jack. He was at around 10% happiness.

Jack was in his 70's and lived in Edinburgh. He had a lot of physical difficulties resulting in his being confined to a wheelchair. He lived alone in a flat and had various home helps to attend to his personal needs.

One day, there was a knock at the door and Jack angrily asked who it was disturbing him. Susan explained that she was from the local hospice and that she had left an envelope the week before and had came back to collect it. There was an initial angry tirade from Jack, but Susan stood her ground, didn't lose her temper and quietly kept talking.

She had been in situations before where people had slammed the door in her face or had shouted at her but this was a new challenge where she was talking to someone behind a closed door. Her persistence paid off and the door slowly opened.

# THE MIND

Jack was taken aback by what he saw; here was a lady with a broad smile actually showing him some real compassion. Jack invited her into his lounge and they sat and chatted for some time about his life and how he felt about the future. Eventually, it was time to go and Susan left with her donation. By the end of the visit something had begun to happen. Jack's attitude to his situation in life was beginning to change.

The next day the home help arrived. As usual the carer was filled with trepidation as she put the key in the door since Jack usually shouted at her over some minor imperfection. As the carer entered the flat she realised right away something was different. The flat seemed warmer and lighter, and was that music she was hearing? When she entered the lounge she noticed it was tidier than usual and when Jack turned round he almost managed a smile. What had happened? Jack, with Susan's help had made a choice. He had made a choice to move from 10% happiness to 20%.

Jack still had all his physical difficulties but he decided to alter the way he felt about them. Things then started to happen. His neighbour, having heard that Jack wasn't actually the disagreeable gentleman that he portrayed, called in to offer him some soup and asked whether he would like to challenge him to a game of chess. This then led to the tenant's association asking if he could be their secretary. Suddenly, Jack was so busy he didn't have time to dwell on the problems he had in his own life.

In this simple story Susan reflected a positive attitude towards Jack. This in turn had affected Jack's feelings about his own life and finally that had affected his relationship with others such as his neighbour.

We all have a choice to make about how we feel about a situation. Our attitude to life has a profound bearing as to how we feel and the level of happiness we experience every day.

Do you have something right now in your life that is affecting your happiness that, if you made a different choice, could affect things positively?

This leads on to those who have a purpose in life. We all know someone who is 30 going on 70 and the converse, someone who is older yet appears much younger.

# THE MIND

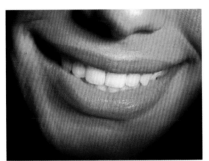

Sarah and Pat were two sisters who had both lost their husbands and were sharing a flat. They began to realise that it was becoming more difficult to attend to their own cooking and general personal care. Having talked it over with their families, they each decided to go into residential accommodation. Sarah's family was in Stirling so she chose a home in that area whereas Pat wanted to be beside her daughter in the borders.

Sarah very soon took charge of this stage in her life by forming a residents committee in her new home. This committee had, as its remit, the right to decide items such as the menu of the day, who should come to entertain them and what outings should be arranged. Sarah was thoroughly enjoying her new role so much that her family hardly saw her. Pat on the other hand was in a home where all the residents sat in the lounge staring at a TV screen.

Who do you think had less illness and lived longer? Yes, it was Sarah of course. So you don't need to be Nelson Mandela or Mother Theresa to have a purpose in life. (It's also interesting the age in which these two well-known individuals were when their outstanding contribution to the world was recognised.) We've all heard of individuals taking up quite adventurous hobbies well into their retirement.

When you have a purpose in life, you are excited and vibrant. You certainly feel better than when you think your life is following a very mundane path.

Have you got a purpose in life? It could be to be the best at what you do at work, or maybe it's to be the best mother, grandfather, sister or brother you can be. Have a purpose and feel better.

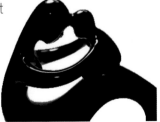

# THE MIND

It is known that the mind can also have a bearing on healing, and the effect in medicine-- and perhaps more significantly in the proven beneficial effects of homeopathy-- is an example of this.

The placebo effect is where a substance containing no active ingredient produces a positive result. A homeopathic medicine is prepared by a series of dilutions and successions (this is where the diluted product is shaken vigorously). This vigorous shaking adds kinetic energy to the solution and the more dilute the preparation, the stronger it becomes. Eventually, the dilution is so great, that not one molecule of the original substance remains. It is difficult to comprehend why these substances work so well for some people.

Could it be that the practitioner plays an important role in the healing process and transmits this will to his patient?

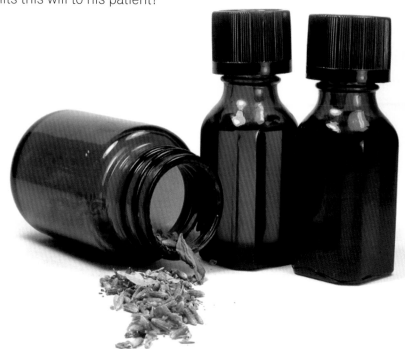

# THE MIND

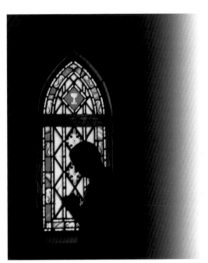

I have witnessed the power of communal prayer in a church setting and also attended a workshop on healing using direction of thought.

The workshop on healing was run by Richard Lawrence in London. We were asked to sit upright in our chairs, close our eyes and imagine a white light coming down through our heads and arms emerging from our bodies through our fingertips. Most of us felt a heat in the palms of our hands. The healer then asked for three individuals to sit at the front facing the group. They were to have some physical discomfort, painful backs or shoulders particularly due to stress. We then held up our hands and sent, as one, a healing force towards the subjects.

At the end of the session, we held our hands aloft and made a slicing motion in order to "cut off" any lasting connection with the problems of these individuals.

The three people stated that they had experienced an improvement in their symptoms after the exercise and the next day several more reports were announced by the chairman of the conference as to the beneficial effects many people had felt.

I have personally felt that healing experience from a group of people and it is an awesome force, which, if you have a spiritual belief, makes you realise what healing power is available to us.

But what about stimulating the part of the mind that is still fresh and young?

Have you ever been on a cruise or indeed a holiday that encompassed new things to do and see? To remain young at heart you must cultivate a mind of curiosity, enthusiasm and dynamism.

# THE MIND

I like to use the example of the pleasure cruise where there are new places to visit almost daily. One of the interesting things to do is to mingle with the locals and learn about their environment and culture. On ship, the entertainment crew arranges frivolous as well as serious activities. Learn how to dance like John Travolta or discover the history of places you are likely to encounter on the way.

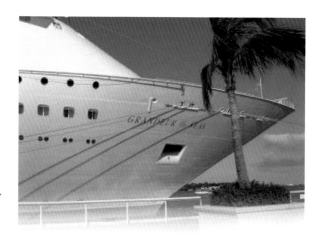

You feel better when you have an enthusiastic mind. You want to learn and are constantly questioning to gain a better understanding. Life is never boring.

If we continue with the analogy of the cruise ship, then behind it being towed is an old battered barge. It is dark and dingy and there are some people who spend their life on the barge rather than the cruise ship.

They polish it relentlessly, carrying with them a lot of baggage from the past. It could be they haven't spoken to a member of their family for years or are harbouring a grudge that they keep stored within their heart. If they only knew this can hold them back in so many ways.

You can never achieve your full potential unless you sort out these issues. It's the same with people who live in a clutter. Whether it's the garage or rooms in your house, loft or car, that clutter is influencing your mind. If you have an unresolved problem or part of your affairs or physical surroundings are in a mess, clear them up. What happens then? You will immediately feel better, your mind will feel lighter and you will be better able to cope with day-to-day living.

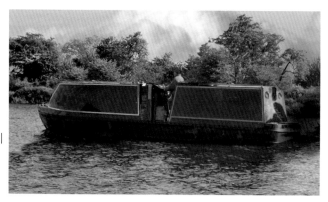

# THE MIND

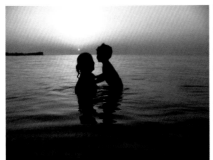

You may have heard the story of the two Tibetan monks who were tracking by foot between villages. They came across a stream where a woman was standing, unable to cross on her own. She pleaded with the monks to carry her over the water and, despite the fact that the monks' order forbade them to touch a woman, the younger man carried her to the other side.

One hour later, the older monk could no longer contain his rage and berated the younger man saying, " how could you carry that woman across the stream?" The younger monk replied simply, "I put that woman down an hour ago, you still carry her on your back."

We all have baggage from the past. When our mind is relieved of that heavy burden, we can resume our enthusiasm for life. A mind that is full of enthusiasm is a youthful mind.

The mind must be allowed to relax. We need to stop the chatter in our heads from time to time and be still. Some people manage this with prayer or a quiet time in church but for others it is meditation. Many people have never experienced a truly quiet moment.

When we realise what it means to be "present in the moment" neither living in the past nor worried about the future, then I feel that true contentment can be experienced.

Illustrate the power of the present with the help of the humble sultana. Go and get one and just hold it in your hand. Look at its myriad of undulations and the rich colour of its skin. Smell the sultana--doesn't it have a wonderful sweet fragrance? Now, put it in your mouth and very slowly suck it, relishing every nuance of taste as it slowly dissolves.

# THE MIND

Do you see how important the present is and how much more appreciative we are of everyday events if we take the time to rediscover simple pleasures?

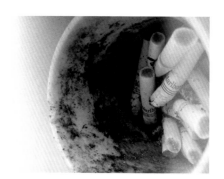

Visualisation and affirmation are useful tools to train the mind in a new habit or way of thinking. If you happen to be a smoker wishing to give up the habit, then I suggest you write on a card the words " I am a non smoker." Equally, if you want to lose weight, then you should write "I only eat nutritious foods."

These affirmations are both positive rather than negative examples. The card should be made up in triplicate and posted on the bathroom mirror, in the car and in a purse or wallet.

Every day you need to say out loud your affirmation dozens of times until the brain relearns the new habit. Take some time also to close your eyes and visualise yourself as a non-smoker with a clear skin or being exactly the right weight wearing those clothes that didn't fit before.

As Ralph Waldo Emerson said, " You become what you think about all day long." If you focus on the negative such as— -" why am I so depressed?" or "why do I feel unloved?" then you immediately find examples to endorse these ideas and so the feeling becomes stronger. If on the other hand you say, " How can I become happy within myself and loveable to others?" then the mind will start to look for solutions. The smoker who says, "I am a non smoker" must reinforce the affirmation with all the reasons why he should stop. Saving money, better health, and social reasons--so many reasons that he feels there is only one way ahead. I can think of lots of reasons why someone might want to lose weight. If that applies to you go ahead and write down a list. The more emotion you put into your list the more likely you are to carry the goal through.

# THE MIND

Visualising a happy event can immediately change the way you feel. Right now, think back to a wonderful time in your life that gave you genuine happiness. Feel how that feels and realise you can reproduce that feeling just by focusing your mind.
Keep asking yourself--" what is great in my life right now?"--focus on it and you will feel better and will even contribute to others happiness around you.

You also need to consider if you have balance in your life in order to be happier and feel better. If you work all the time without giving due consideration to families and friends then you may find yourself on your own wondering what happened. A balance is also needed in terms of recreational pursuits. If you are an accountant, then take up Latin American dancing rather than the stock market as your hobby.

**Step 10 - The mind is a powerful tool. Use it wisely.**

# NOW WHAT!

**Now that you have read the book, and you want to look better, feel better and live a better life, follow the steps.**

Step 1 – Create a fantastic life with the Star of Life-Life Plan.

Step 2 – Get more oxygen into your body.

Step 3 – Consume more water on a daily basis.

Step 4 – Make a nutritious diet your way of life.

Step 5 – Consider taking nutritional supplements.

Step 6 – Get moving.

Step 7 – Reduce the toxins in your body.

Step 8 – Get your relationships in order.

Step 9 – Get yourself some quality sleep

Step 10 – The mind is a powerful tool. Use it wisely.

## *Live your life to the full*

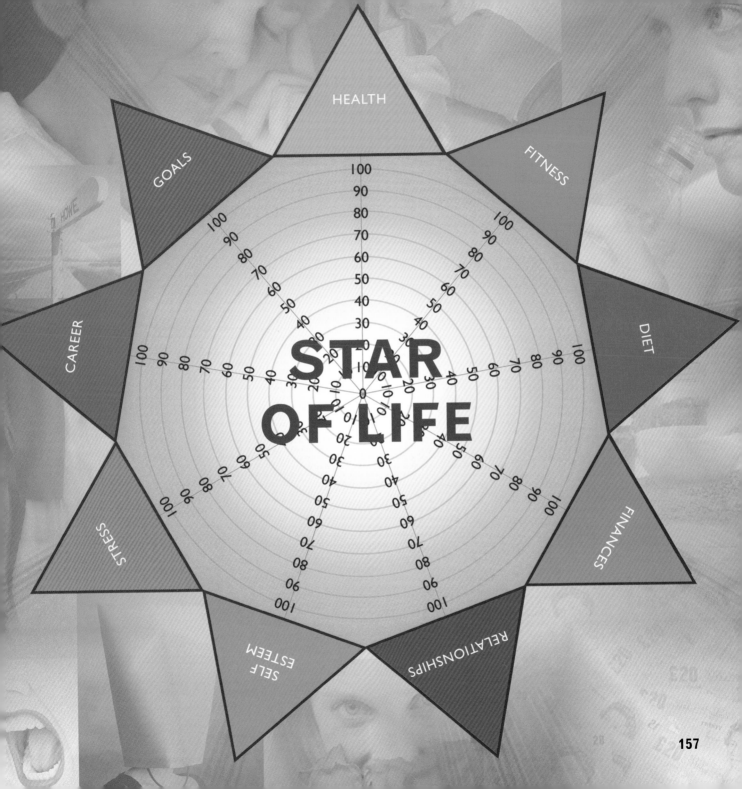

STAR
OF LIFE

HEALTH

FITNESS

DIET

FINANCES

RELATIONSHIPS

SELF ESTEEM

STRESS

CAREER

GOALS

AFTER

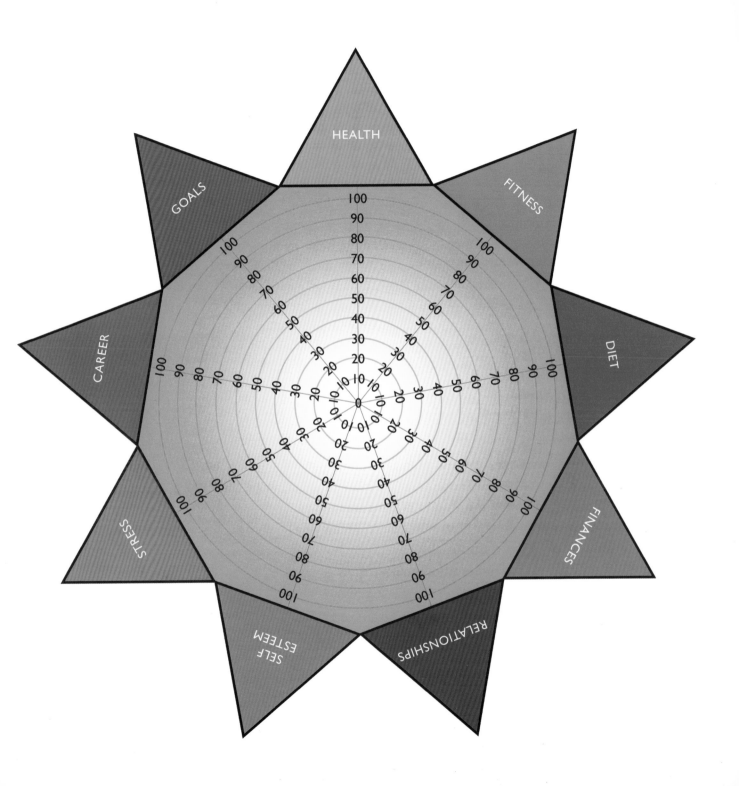

# FURTHER INFORMATION

**Rebounder Agent**
**Nutritional supplements**
**Live Blood Microscopy**
**Toxin free personal care products**
**Flaxseed oil products**
**The Detox Brush**
**Detox Products**
**Wrist Pulse Meter**
**Reverse Osmosis**
**Network Marketing**
**Green alkalising drinks**
**UDO's Oil Omega 3, 6 and 9**

...all at www.newlifehealthcare.co.uk

**Yoga instruction www.chiyogacentre.com**
**Swiss Ball instruction\stockist ssb2441@hotmail.com, 00 44 (0) 7862 222 672**
**Anthony Robbins Unleash the Power Within weekends**
**George Parnerou 0207 351 91—Ext 608 (London Link line)**
**Sovereign Singing  Edwin Coppard**
**The Silva Method www.silvamethod.co.uk**
**Detox for Life Loree Taylor Jordan**
**100% Health  Patrick Holford**
**Rebounding for Health Margaret Hawkins**

The author, Elizabeth Roddick is available for presentations.
For details please contact Focus Marketing at murefocus@lineone.net

**If you would like to experience life coaching on any aspect of the Star of Life then contact Elizabeth at elizabeth@newlifehealthcare.co.uk**